# The Complete SAQ Study Guide

## Medicine, surgery and the clinical specialties

*Edited by*

**ANDREW SCHOFIELD**
MBChB DRCOG
*Senior House Officer*
*University Hospitals of Leicester NHS Trust*

*and*

**PAUL SCHOFIELD**
MBChB MRCGP MRCP DCH DFSRH
*General Practitioner*
*Cambridgeshire*

Radcliffe Publishing
London • New York

**Radcliffe Publishing Ltd**
St Mark's House
Sheperdess Walk
London N1 7BQ
United Kingdom

**www.radcliffehealth.com**

British Library Cataloguing in Publication Data

A catalogue record for this book is available from the British Library.

ISBN-13: 978 184619 579 2

The paper used for the text pages of this book is FSC® certified. FSC (The Forest Stewardship Council®) is an international network to promote responsible management of the world's forests.

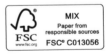

MIX
Paper from responsible sources
FSC® C013056

Typeset by Darkriver Design, Auckland, New Zealand
Printed and bound by TJI Digital, Padstow, Cornwall, UK

# Contents

# Preface

As a medical student, I found there was a major lack in short-answer question (SAQ) books that covered all of the topics that any medical school curriculum would include. So when my housemate (James Baldock) and I were revising for any of our clinical attachment exams and finals, we decided to write our own SAQs to help us. This sparked an idea to write a more detailed and fully encompassing set of questions. So I gained the help of my other colleagues – Scott, Michael and James, who all did really well throughout medical school – to help me write the material, as well as asking my brother (who has got 7 years more experience than any of us) to help edit.

The book covers 20 separate subject areas, each having 10 or so questions covering the major topics. The answers also include a topic summary to incorporate any part of that topic we felt was important but not mentioned in the questions. As well as this, there is a practice paper section that you can use in order to test yourself under exam conditions. However, this book is not designed to be a replacement for a detailed textbook, and I would recommend any of the Radcliffe Publishing textbooks as a source for note-taking and building a foundation of knowledge. Also, it is important to remember, nothing replaces getting clinical experience on the wards!

Finally, I wish any medical student using this book the best of luck in their medical school exams.

**Andrew Schofield**
*March 2012*

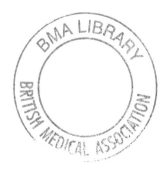

# List of contributors

**James Baldock** MBChB
Senior House Officer
Oxford University Hospitals NHS Trust

**Scott Mabbutt** MBChB
Senior House Officer
Bundaberg Base Hospital, Australia

**Michael Bowen** MBChB (Hons)
Honorary Clinical Educator
FY2 in Emergency Medicine
University Hospitals of Leicester NHS Trust

**James Dearman** MBChB (Hons)
Honorary Clinical Educator
FY2 in Emergency Medicine
University Hospitals of Leicester NHS Trust

# List of abbreviations

| | |
|---|---|
| AAA | Abdominal aortic aneurysm |
| AACG | Acute angle-closure glaucoma |
| A&E | Accident and emergency |
| ABC | Airway, breathing, circulation |
| $ABCD_2$ | Age, blood pressure, clinical features, duration of symptoms, diabetes |
| ABCDE | Chest X-ray: Air, bones (clavicles), cardiovascular, diaphragm, extra |
| ABCDE | Melanoma: Asymmetry, border, colour, diameter and evolution |
| ABCDE | Resuscitation: Airway, breathing, circulation, disability and exposure |
| ABG | Arterial blood gas |
| ACE | Angiotensin-converting enzyme |
| ACEi | Angiotensin-converting enzyme inhibitor |
| ACS | Acute coronary syndrome |
| ACTH | Adrenocorticotropic hormone |
| ADH | Vasopressin |
| AF | Atrial fibrillation |
| AFP | Alpha-fetoprotein |
| AIDS | Acquired immune deficiency syndrome |
| ALP | Alkaline phosphatase |
| ALT | Alanine transaminase |
| AMTS | Abbreviated mental test score |
| ANA | Anti-nuclear antibody |
| ANCA | Anti-neutrophil cytoplasmic antibody |
| anti-dsDNA | Anti-double-stranded DNA |
| AP | Anteroposterior |
| APLS | Antiphospholipid syndrome |
| APTT | Activated partial thromboplastin time |
| ARDS | Acute respiratory distress syndrome |
| ARMD | Age-related macular degeneration |
| AST | Aspartate aminotransferase |

| | |
|---|---|
| AVM | Arteriovenous malformation |
| $\beta_2$ | Beta-2 |
| BCC | Basal cell carcinoma |
| BCG | Bacillus Calmette-Guérin |
| BiPAP | Bi-level positive airway pressure |
| BMI | Body mass index |
| BP | Blood pressure |
| BPH | Benign prostatic hyperplasia |
| BPPV | Benign paroxysmal positional vertigo |
| BTS | British Thoracic Society |
| C3 | Complement factor 3 |
| CABG | Coronary artery bypass graft |
| CAM | Confusion Assessment Method |
| CAP | Community-acquired pneumonia |
| CBD | Common bile duct |
| CBT | Cognitive behavioural therapy |
| CCB | Calcium channel blocker |
| CCP | Cyclic citrullinated protein |
| CCU | Coronary care unit |
| CF | Cystic fibrosis |
| CIN | Cervical intraepithelial neoplasia |
| CJD | Creutzfeldt-Jakob disease |
| CK | Creatine kinase |
| CKD | Chronic kidney disease |
| CK-MB | Creatine kinase muscle and brain isoenzyme |
| CML | Chronic myeloid leukaemia |
| CNS | Central nervous system |
| CNV | Choroidal neovascularisation |
| COCP | Combined oral contraceptive pill |
| COPD | Chronic obstructive pulmonary disease |
| CPAP | Continuous positive airway pressure |
| CRP | C-reactive protein |
| CSF | Cerebrospinal fluid |
| CT | Computed tomography |
| CTG | Cardiotocography |
| CTPA | Computed tomography pulmonary angiogram |
| CVS | Cardiovascular system |
| CXR | Chest X-ray |

| | |
|---|---|
| DC | Direct current |
| DEXA | Dual-energy X-ray absorptiometry |
| DI | Diabetes insipidus |
| DIC | Disseminated intravascular coagulation |
| DMARD | Disease-modifying antirheumatic drug |
| DSH | Deliberate self-harm |
| DVLA | Driver and Vehicle Licensing Authority |
| DVT | Deep vein thrombosis |
| EBV | Epstein-Barr virus |
| ECG | Electrocardiogram |
| eGFR | Estimated glomerular filtration rate |
| ENT | Ear, nose and throat |
| ERCP | Endoscopic retrograde cholangiopancreatography |
| ESBL | Extended-spectrum beta-lactamase |
| ESR | Erythrocyte sedimentation rate |
| ETT | Exercise tolerance test |
| EVAR | Endovascular aneurysm repair |
| FAST | Focused assessment with sonography for trauma |
| FBC | Full blood count |
| $Fe^{2+}$ | Iron |
| $FEV_1$ | Forced expiratory volume (in 1 second) |
| FSH | Follicle-stimulating hormone |
| FVC | Functional vital capacity |
| G6PD | Glucose-6-phosphate dehydrogenase |
| GA | General anaesthesia |
| GCS | Glasgow Coma Score |
| GI | Gastrointestinal |
| GnRH | Gonadotropin-releasing hormone |
| GOJ | Gastro-oesophageal junction |
| GORD | Gastro-oesophageal reflux disease |
| GTN | Glyceryl trinitrate |
| HACEK | *Haemophilus, Actinobacillus, Cardiobacterium, Eikenella, Kingella* |
| HADS | Hospital Anxiety and Depression Scale |
| Hb F | Foetal haemoglobin |
| HbSAg | Hepatitis B surface antigen |
| hCG | Human chorionic gonadotropin |
| HHV | Human herpes virus |
| HIV | Human immunodeficiency virus |
| HNPCC | Hereditary non-polyposis colorectal cancer |

| | |
|---|---|
| HR | Heart rate |
| HSP | Henoch–Schönlein purpura |
| IBS | Irritable bowel syndrome |
| IGF-1 | Insulin-like growth factor 1 |
| Igs | Immunoglobulins |
| IHD | Ischaemic heart disease |
| ILD | Interstitial lung disease |
| INR | International normalised ratio |
| IRDS | Infant respiratory distress syndrome |
| ITP | Immune thrombocytopenic purpura |
| ITU | Intensive treatment unit |
| IUCD | Intrauterine contraceptive device |
| IVDU | Intravenous drug user |
| JVP | Jugular venous pressure |
| kPa | Kilopascal |
| KUB | Kidney, ureter and bladder |
| LCP | Liverpool Care Pathway |
| LDH | Lactate dehydrogenase |
| LFT | Liver function test |
| LH | Luteinising hormone |
| LHRH | Luteinising hormone-releasing hormone |
| LLETZ | Large loop excision of the transition zone |
| LMWH | Low molecular weight heparin |
| LRTI | Lower respiratory tract infection |
| LTOT | Long-term oxygen therapy |
| LUTS | Lower urinary tract symptoms |
| MC&S | Microscopy, culture & sensitivities |
| MCH | Mean corpuscular haemoglobin |
| MCV | Mean corpuscular volume |
| MEN | Multiple endocrine neoplasia |
| MGUS | Monoclonal gammopathy of undeterimined significance |
| MI | Myocardial infarction |
| MPS | Myocardial perfusion scintigraphy |
| MRI | Magnetic resonance imaging |
| MSU | Mid-stream urine collection |
| NA | Noradrenaline |
| NAC | N-acetylcysteine |
| NAPQI | N-acetyl-p-benzoquinone imine |

| | |
|---|---|
| NICE | National Institute for Health and Clinical Excellence |
| NIV | Non-invasive ventilation |
| NSAIDs | Non-steroidal anti-inflammatory drugs |
| NSTEMI | Non-ST-segment elevation myocardial infarction |
| O$_2$ sats | Oxygen saturations |
| OCD | Obsessive-compulsive disorder |
| OCP | Oral contraceptive pill |
| OCSP | Oxford Community Stroke Project |
| OCT | Optical coherence tomography |
| OGD | Oesophagogastroduodenoscopy |
| OGTT | Oral glucose tolerance test |
| PAN | Polyarteritis nodosa |
| PaO$_2$ | Partial pressure of oxygen |
| PCA | Patient-controlled analgesia |
| PCI | Percutaneous intervention |
| PCOS | Polycystic ovarian syndrome |
| PDA | Patent ductus arteriosus |
| PE | Pulmonary embolism |
| PEF | Peak expiratory flow |
| PET | Positron emission tomography |
| PID | Pelvic inflammatory disease |
| PMH | Past medical history |
| PND | Paroxysmal nocturnal dyspnoea |
| POP | Progesterone-only pill |
| PPH | Post-partum haemorrhage |
| PPI | Proton pump inhibitor |
| PPV | Positive predictive value |
| PR | Per-rectal |
| PRN | *Pro re nata* |
| PSA | Prostate-specific antigen |
| PTH | Parathyroid hormone |
| RA | Rheumatoid arthritis |
| RCC | Renal cell carcinoma |
| RR | Respiratory rate |
| SAH | Subarachnoid haemorrhage |
| SCC | Squamous cell carcinoma |
| SHO | Senior house officer |
| SIADH | Syndrome of inappropriate ADH secretion |

| | |
|---|---|
| SIRS | Systemic inflammatory response syndrome |
| SLE | Systemic lupus erythematosus |
| SNRI | Serotonin-norepinephrine reuptake inhibitor |
| SSRI | Selective serotonin reuptake inhibitor |
| STEMI | ST-segment elevation myocardial infarction |
| STI | Sexually transmitted infection |
| SUFE | Slipped upper femoral epiphysis |
| TACI | Total anterior circulation infarc |
| TCC | Transitional cell carcinoma |
| TED | Thromboembolic deterrent |
| TFT | Thyroid function test |
| TIA | Transient ischaemic attack |
| TNF-$\alpha$ | Tumour necrosis factor-alpha |
| TNM | Tumour, node, metastasis |
| TORCH | Toxoplasmosis, other infections, rubella, cytomegalovirus, herpes simplex virus-2 |
| TRUS | Transrectal ultrasound |
| TSH | Thyroid-stimulating hormone |
| TTP | Thrombotic thrombocytopenic purpura |
| TURBT | Transurethral resection of bladder tumour |
| TURP | Transurethral resection of the prostate |
| TVT | Transvaginal tape |
| $TxA_2$ | Thromboxine |
| U&E | Urea and electrolytes |
| USS | Ultrasound scan |
| UTI | Urinary tract infection |
| VEGF | Vascular endothelial growth factor |
| VF | Ventricular fibrillation |
| VSD | Ventricular septal defect |
| VT | Ventricular tachycardia |
| VTE | Venous thromboembolism |
| WCC | White cell count |

# Medicine

# Cardiology

**Q1**  A 68-year-old man presents to A&E with a 20-minute history of severe left-sided chest pain. Following an ECG, you spot ST elevation in the anterior leads and diagnose an anterior STEMI.

1. Give four risk factors for ischaemic heart disease. **(2)**
2. Which artery supplies the anterior territory of the myocardium? **(1)**
3. Give three aspects of your immediate management plan. **(3)**
4. What two management options are available to treat his STEMI? **(2)**
5. Give four medications that may be started prior to discharge. **(2)**

**Q2**  A 68-year-old retired man with known angina is admitted to hospital via ambulance with central chest pain. An ECG reveals ST elevation in the lateral leads, and he is immediately taken to the cardiac catheterisation lab for a primary PCI.

1. Name the leads on a 12-lead ECG in which you would expect to see ST elevation. **(1)**
2. Which vessel is likely to be affected? **(1)**
3. Give two cardiac enzymes that commonly rise following cardiac damage. **(2)**
4. He is discharged the following week. Give two abnormalities that may be seen on his ECG prior to discharge. **(2)**
5. The patient asks whether it is safe for him to drive. What would you tell him? **(1)**
6. Give three possible complications of coronary angiography. **(3)**

**Q3** A 58-year-old man visits his GP with a heavy, central chest pain that he has noticed over the past few months. It is usually brought on when walking the dog, causing him to stop and sit down for 5 minutes. The pain then settles and he is able to walk home slowly. His wife is concerned about the pain and has encouraged him to see a doctor. He is diagnosed with angina. His GP starts aspirin, arranges for blood tests and refers him to cardiology for further investigation.

1. Other than exertion, give two possible triggers of angina. **(2)**
2. Give two other symptoms he may experience during an episode of angina. **(1)**
3. Name two blood tests that his GP may have requested and why. **(2)**
4. Name three other tests that may be used to investigate angina. **(3)**
5. How does aspirin reduce the risk of coronary events? **(2)**

**Q4** A 74-year-old man has a significant history of ischaemic heart disease and is brought into A&E resus severely short of breath and complaining of central chest pain. You suspect he is having an MI and has acute pulmonary oedema.

1. Give three signs of acute pulmonary oedema you would look for on examination. **(3)**
2. Following your initial assessment, give four investigations you would request. **(2)**
3. Name two drugs that may be used in the treatment of acute pulmonary oedema. **(2)**

Following the treatment you initiate, he improves greatly and his MI was managed medically. The following day, you request numerous blood tests, including biochemistry, and he is found to be hypokalaemic ($K^+$ 3.1).

4. Name one drug that may have been used that can cause hypokalaemia. **(1)**
5. Give two ways you could raise his potassium medically. **(2)**

**5** You are called urgently to the cardiology ward to see a 74-year-old man being treated medically for an NSTEMI 2 days previously. He has been complaining of chest pain for the past 10 minutes, similar to the pain he had when admitted to hospital. The nurse has given him some GTN, but the pain persists. The nurse has taken an ECG, which reveals ST elevation in leads II, III and aVF with reciprocal changes elsewhere.

1. Which territory of the myocardium do leads II, III and aVF represent? **(1)**
2. Which vessel is responsible for this territory? **(1)**

You initiate treatment for a STEMI and call your seniors to inform them when the nurse calls for you to come back urgently as he has stopped breathing. A quick assessment confirms he has stopped breathing and his pulse is no longer palpable.

3. Give two things you would do next. **(2)**

The crash team arrive and the patient is connected to the defibrillator. His ECG shows a regular rhythm at a rate of approximately 140 bpm, broad QRS complexes and an occasional capture beat.

4. What is the normal QRS interval? **(1)**
5. What is a capture beat? **(1)**
6. Name the rhythm disturbance. **(1)**
7. Is this a shockable rhythm? **(1)**
8. Give two drugs that may be used during the arrest. **(2)**

**6** An 86-year-old man has known congestive cardiac failure secondary to hypertension.

1. What system is used to classify the severity of heart failure? **(1)**
2. Give three symptoms of left ventricular failure. **(3)**
3. Give three signs of heart failure on a chest radiograph. **(3)**
4. Specifically, how and where does furosemide act? **(2)**
5. The above patient is admitted to hospital with worsening confusion and is treated for a UTI. His admission ECG reveals a reverse tick pattern, ST depression and T-wave inversion in V5–V6. What drug often used in heart failure causes this? **(1)**

**Q7** A 52-year-old white British man attends his GP surgery concerned he may have high blood pressure as his younger brother has recently been started on medication for this. He smokes 20 cigarettes a day and has done for 30 years, and also tells you his father died of a heart attack aged 62. On examination, he is 173 cm tall and weighs 97.5 kg. His blood pressure is 166/94. You ask him to come back 1 week later for another blood pressure check. This time, his blood pressure is 160/92. You decide to start medication for hypertension.

1. Calculate his BMI. **(1)**
2. How would you classify his BMI? **(1)**
3. Give three pieces of lifestyle advice you would recommend. **(3)**
4. What class of drug would be first-line in this man to treat hypertension? **(1)**
5. Give two side effects you would make the patient aware of prior to starting this medication. **(2)**
6. Give two signs that may be visible on the retina of someone with hypertensive retinopathy. **(2)**

**Q8** A normally fit and well 72-year-old lady attends a health screening clinic at her GP surgery. Her blood pressure is found to be 172/88, her cholesterol is 5.9, random glucose is 5.0 and urinalysis is normal. An appointment is booked for her to see her GP, and her blood pressure is 168/92. She has no family history of cardiovascular disease and takes no regular medications. She is started on bendroflumethiazide for hypertension and simvastatin for hypercholesterolaemia.

1. What class of drug is now considered first-line in this age group? **(1)**
2. Give three complications of essential hypertension. **(3)**
3. What is the mechanism of action of simvastatin? **(2)**
4. Give two signs of hypercholesterolaemia you may find on examination. **(2)**
5. The same patient returns 2 days later with severe pain in the big toe on her right foot. On examination, it is red, swollen and tender to palpation. What is the most likely diagnosis? **(1)**
6. Name one drug you may use to treat the acute phase of this condition. **(1)**

**9** You are the house officer on the emergency admissions unit. You are asked to see a 76-year-old male who is complaining of palpitations. When you examine the patient, you notice he has an irregular pulse.

1. What is the most likely diagnosis? **(1)**
2. Name three common causes of your answer above. **(3)**
3. The nurse shows you an ECG that was done on arrival. Name two features you expect to find on the ECG. **(2)**
4. Name two other symptoms the patient may be complaining of. **(1)**
5. Your consultant says that cardioversion is the best treatment in this patient. Name two methods that could be used to cardiovert the patient. **(1)**
6. Name two medications that may be used long-term in this patient if cardioversion fails. **(1)**
7. Name two complications of the condition you have diagnosed. **(1)**

**10** A 45-year-old man is admitted via A&E, having been unwell for 1–2 weeks. He had initially been feeling hot and cold, but has now developed night sweats and worsening shortness of breath. On examination, he is febrile at 38.5, tachycardic at 140 bpm reg, RR 24, BP 146/58, O$_2$ sats 95% on air. Examination of the heart reveals a high-pitched, early diastolic murmur. Course crepitations are heard at the lung bases. You suspect infective endocarditis.

1. Outline your immediate management plan. **(3)**
2. Which organism is commonly responsible for infective endocarditis? **(1)**
3. The staff nurse is asked to dip his urine sample. Why? **(1)**
4. Examining of the fundi reveals a boat-shaped retinal haemorrhage with a pale centre. What is this called? **(1)**
5. What criteria are used to make a diagnosis of infective endocarditis? **(1)**
6. Other than an early diastolic murmur, give three signs of aortic regurgitation. **(3)**

**Q11** A 23-year-old lady is admitted by her GP with worsening shortness of breath, high fevers and suspected infective endocarditis. She is an IV drug user, and has been unwell for 6 days. She is febrile, tachycardic and hypotensive. A pansystolic murmur is heard at the lower sternal edge when she inspires. There is also a right ventricular heave and her liver is pulsatile and enlarged. Bloods reveal raised neutrophils and raised inflammatory markers.

1. Given the above history, what valve disease caused the endocarditis? **(1)**
2. Which organism is most likely to be responsible in this case? **(1)**
3. How should blood cultures be taken? **(3)**
4. Other than blood tests, give two further investigations you would request. **(2)**
5. Other than IV drug users, give two examples of pre-existing cardiac disease that increases the risk of patients developing endocarditis. **(2)**
6. What can be done in these patients to help prevent endocarditis? **(1)**

# Respiratory

Q1 A 24-year-old man has suffered with asthma and other 'atopic conditions' since his early childhood. He uses a salbutamol inhaler when required and maximum dose of inhaled beclometasone twice daily. He visits his GP with a worsening dry cough, increased use of his salbutamol inhaler and poor sleep.

1. Give four common triggers of asthma. **(4)**
2. What pattern is seen on spirometry in asthmatics? **(1)**
3. How can asthma be diagnosed using spirometry? **(1)**
4. His GP concludes his asthma is poorly controlled and initiates another drug. What class of drug should be started next according to BTS guidelines? **(1)**
5. Give two other 'atopic conditions' he may suffer from. **(2)**
6. Specifically, how does salbutamol improve symptoms in asthmatics? **(1)**

**Q2** A 62-year-old man has chronic obstructive pulmonary disease (COPD), has smoked 30 cigarettes a day since he was 14 and is adamant he won't quit. He is on maximal treatment, and his respiratory consultant has discussed long-term oxygen therapy (LTOT) on numerous occasions.

1. For how many pack-years has he smoked? **(1)**
2. What pattern will spirometry show? **(1)**
3. What physiological measurement is used to determine the severity of COPD? **(1)**

He is admitted to hospital with fever, dyspnoea, productive cough and green sputum and is treated for an infective exacerbation of COPD. You request blood tests, a chest X-ray and take an arterial blood gas on air. The results are:

| | | |
|---|---|---|
| pH | 7.26 | (7.35–7.45) |
| pCO$_2$ | 9.7 kPa | (> 10.6) |
| pO$_2$ | 6.7 kPa | (4.7–6) |
| Bicarb | 24 mmol/L | (22–28) |

4. Give two abnormalities seen on the above blood gas result. **(2)**
5. What implications does this have on oxygen therapy and why? **(2)**
6. You diagnose an infective exacerbation of COPD. Other than oxygen, give four aspects of your subsequent management plan. **(2)**
7. Why is LTOT not appropriate for this patient currently? **(1)**

**3** A 74-year-old lady presents to the acute medical admissions unit with a 3-day history of worsening shortness of breath, productive cough and fever. Her past medical history includes hypertension and high cholesterol, for which she takes atenolol, ramipril and simvastatin.

On examination, she has a temperature of 38.4, HR 118 bpm reg, BP 96/64, RR 24, $O_2$ sats 94%, heart sounds are normal and she has signs of consolidation in the left lower lobe. Her AMTS is 9/10. Blood tests on admission include Hb 11.3, WCC 18.12, Neut 16.34, Plts 356, Na 142, K 4.8, urea 8.4, creatinine 114 and CRP 114.5. Her LFTs are normal. You diagnose community-acquired pneumonia.

1. Give two signs on examination of consolidation. **(2)**
2. Give two further tests you would arrange at this stage. **(2)**
3. What is her CURB-65 score (show how you came to this score)? **(2)**
4. Give the three most likely organisms to cause CAP. **(3)**
5. You start amoxicillin and clarithromycin. What alteration will you make to her regular medications whilst she is taking these and why? **(1)**

**4** A 62-year-old man presents via A&E with right-sided pleuritic chest pain that has developed over the past 2–3 days. He has also been feeling more short of breath, has a productive cough, green sputum and has been feeling hot and cold.

1. What further information do you require in order to calculate his CURB-65 score? **(4)**
2. His CURB-65 score is 2. Will he need hospital admission? Explain your answer. **(1)**
3. Give two possible complications of pneumonia. **(2)**
4. Fill in the following table with the chest signs you would expect to see when examining a patient with each of the following chest problems **(3)**

| | Chest expansion | Percussion note | Auscultation |
|---|---|---|---|
| Consolidation | | | |
| Pleural effusion | | | |
| Pneumothorax | | | |

**Q5** A 42-year-old Zimbabwean man is seen in the respiratory clinic and has pulmonary tuberculosis. He had been complaining of shortness of breath and a productive cough. The diagnosis was made following a chest X-ray and staining of his sputum. The consultant starts him on a course of four antibiotics to treat this. TB had been on the decline, but the number of cases worldwide is now rising rapidly.

1. Give two reasons why cases of TB may be on the rise. **(2)**
2. Which antibiotics do you think he will be taking? Indicate the duration of the course for each antibiotic. **(4)**
3. Why are four antibiotics used? **(1)**
4. A few days after his clinic appointment, Mr A attends his GP concerned as he is passing red-orange urine. What is the cause of this? **(1)**
5. A 26-year-old lady, also found to have TB, presents with fever, malaise and painful, purple nodules over her shins. What are these lesions on her shins called? **(1)**
6. Name two other causes of this. **(1)**

**Q6** A 17-year-old lady has cystic fibrosis and is seen in the respiratory clinic regularly, as she has developed bronchiectasis.

1. What is the incidence of cystic fibrosis in the UK? **(1)**
2. What is bronchiectasis? **(2)**
3. Give two organisms that commonly colonise the lungs of those with CF. **(2)**
4. Give three other causes of bronchiectasis. **(3)**
5. Give two complications of bronchiectasis. **(2)**

**Q7** A 68-year-old lady is brought into A&E 10 days following a left total knee replacement complaining of severe central chest pain. The pain came on suddenly at home, and paracetamol and codeine have provided no relief. An arterial blood gas reveals the following: pH 7.42, $pCO_2$ 3.5 kPa, $pO_2$ 7.8 kPa, BE 0.6. You suspect she has a pulmonary embolism.

1. Other than recent surgery, give two risk factors for PE. **(2)**
2. What abnormality is seen on the above ABG? **(1)**
3. What underlying mechanism is responsible for this abnormality? **(1)**
4. Name two investigations that may be requested to confirm the suspected diagnosis. **(2)**

Investigations confirm a PE and the patient is started on low molecular weight heparin and warfarin.

5. What will the target INR range be? **(1)**
6. Given she has never had a DVT or PE previously, how long would you continue warfarin for? **(1)**
7. What measures can be taken to reduce the risk of a DVT/PE developing in patients undergoing a total knee replacement? **(2)**

**Q8** A 68-year-old man has been diagnosed with lung cancer. His GP had treated him for a lower respiratory tract infection that was not improving, so arranged a chest X-ray which revealed a suspicious lesion. Further investigations have confirmed metastatic squamous cell carcinoma.

1.  Other than a non-resolving LRTI/pneumonia, give four symptoms someone with lung cancer may present with. **(2)**
2.  Give three sites that lung cancers are most likely to metastasise to. **(3)**
3.  Other than chest X-ray, name two imaging modalities that may have been used to determine the extent of his disease. **(2)**
4.  What staging system is used for squamous cell carcinoma of the lung? **(1)**

This man presents 2 months later to A&E with worsening shortness of breath, severe headache and swelling of his arms and legs. On examination, he has periorbital oedema, non-pulsatile dilated neck veins and dilated collateral vessels of his arms and chest. You ask him to lift his arms above his head and keep them there for a minute. You notice that he appears slightly blue in the face, his JVP is more raised and he has developed an inspiratory stridor.

5.  What is your diagnosis? **(1)**
6.  What test has been described above? **(1)**

**Q9** A 52-year-old lady is referred to the acute medical team by her GP. She presents with progressive shortness of breath, worse on exertion, a dry cough and weight loss. Examination reveals tachypnoea, finger clubbing and fine end-inspiratory crepitations. Following numerous investigations, she is diagnosed with cryptogenic fibrosing alveolitis (idiopathic pulmonary fibrosis) and is started on steroids.

1. Name two abnormalities that may be seen on her chest radiograph. **(2)**
2. Her lung function was tested using spirometry. Indicate whether the following will be high, normal or low: (a) FVC; (b) $FEV_1$; (c) $FEV_1$ to FVC ratio. **(3)**
3. Extrinsic allergic alveolitis is another cause of pulmonary fibrosis. Give two causes of this. **(2)**
4. Name two non-respiratory causes of pulmonary fibrosis. **(1)**
5. Give two other respiratory causes of clubbing. **(2)**

**Q10** A 54-year-old man visits his GP, complaining of fatigue. He has received a warning at work by his boss, who caught him sleeping at his desk. His wife has put up with his snoring for many years, but has been becoming increasingly concerned that he stops breathing on numerous occasions throughout the night. On examination, he is obese and has a large neck circumference. He is asked to complete a questionnaire.

1. Given the history, what is the most likely diagnosis? **(1)**
2. What questionnaire will he have been asked to complete? **(1)**
3. Other than obesity, give two risk factors for this condition. **(2)**
4. How is this condition diagnosed? **(1)**
5. Give two aspects of the management of this condition. **(2)**

In severe cases, this condition can lead to cor pulmonale.

6. What is cor pulmonale? **(1)**
7. Give one abnormality you may expect to see on a chest radiograph of a patient with cor pulmonale. **(1)**
8. Give one abnormality you may expect to see on an ECG of the same patient. **(1)**

**Q11** A 33-year-old lady was found to have bilateral hilar lymphadenopathy on a chest X-ray, which was part of a septic screen during a recent admission to hospital in which she was treated for pyelonephritis. Following a transbronchial biopsy, she is diagnosed with sarcoidosis and started on prednisolone.

1. Give two other possible causes of bilateral hilar lymphadenopathy. **(2)**
2. What is likely to have been seen on the biopsy? **(1)**
3. Give four extrapulmonary manifestations of sarcoidosis. **(2)**
4. Give two pieces of advice you would give her prior to starting long-term corticosteroids. **(2)**
5. Give six side effects of long-term corticosteroids. **(3)**

Q12 A 57-year-old lady with metastatic ovarian cancer presents with worsening shortness of breath and reduced exercise tolerance. Examination suggests a left sided pleural effusion, and you arrange a chest X-ray to confirm this.

1. Give two signs of a pleural effusion on examination of the chest. **(2)**
2. You watch as your registrar performs a pleural tap. He asks whether he should insert the needle above or below the rib. What is your answer and why? **(2)**

In order to determine the nature of the effusion, the protein and LDH content of the accumulated fluid are measured.

3. Indicate if the protein content is high (> 30 d/L) whether it would it be an exudate or transudate.
4. Indicate if the LDH is high (> 200 IU/L) whether it would be an exudate or transudate.
5. Other than protein content and LDH, name two other tests you would ask the lab to perform on the pleural fluid. **(2)**

The patient's effusion is found to be a malignant pleural effusion. It is drained and she is discharged 3 days following admission. Two weeks later, she returns with the same symptoms, and investigations reveal reaccumulation of the effusion. Your consultant explains to her that they will drain the effusion and then instil a chemical to 'plug the gap'.

6. What procedure is your consultant referring to, and name one substance/chemical that may be used for this? **(2)**

# Renal

Q1 A 56-year-old type 2 diabetic was recently admitted under the general surgeons with lower abdominal pain. No cause for his abdominal pain was found. It was noted, however, that his renal function had deteriorated, having been normal 4 months previously. This was discussed with the renal registrar, who advised a referral to the outpatients' clinic. You are asked to see him in clinic, and his U&Es are as follows: $Na^+$ 139, $K^+$ 5.1, urea 8.8, creatinine 118, eGFR 52.

1. What stage CKD does this man have? **(1)**
2. Other than diabetes, give four common causes of CKD. **(2)**
3. A renal USS is arranged. Give two reasons why this may have been requested. **(2)**
4. He regularly takes metformin, gliclazide and aspirin. Which class of medication is likely to be added? **(1)**
5. Give two common side effects associated with drugs in this class. **(2)**
6. It is important to closely monitor his renal function and diabetic control. Give two other blood tests it is important to check regularly. **(2)**

Mrs T, a 73-year-old lady, is seen regularly by the renal clinic. She has chronic kidney disease and is being readied for renal replacement therapy. Her most recent eGFR is 14 mL/min.

1. What stage CKD does Mrs T have? **(1)**
2. Give three signs of chronic kidney disease you may find on examination. **(3)**
3. Explain the basic principles of haemodialysis. **(2)**
4. Give two complications of peritoneal dialysis. **(2)**

Mrs T opts for renal transplantation and receives a cadaveric kidney. She will be on lifelong immunosuppressants.

5. Organ rejection is a possible complication of renal transplantation. What time period determines whether the organ rejection is acute or chronic? **(1)**
6. Mrs T is now seen annually by a dermatologist. Why is this? **(1)**

 Mr C, a 74-year-old man, has stage 4 chronic kidney disease, and recent blood tests have shown low calcium and a high PTH.

1. What form of hyperparathyroidism is this? **(1)**
2. Give two actions of PTH. **(2)**
3. At what two sites does hydroxylation of vitamin D occur? **(2)**
4. What is the term given to bone disease in patients with renal failure? **(1)**
5. Give two aspects of the management of this condition. **(2)**

Mr C's blood tests are repeated the following year and show tertiary hyperparathyroidism.

6. Indicate whether you would expect the calcium to be high, low or normal. **(1)**
7. Indicate whether you would expect the PTH to be high, low or normal. **(1)**
8. Why has this developed? **(1)**

Q4 A 72-year-old man is admitted via A&E with worsening confusion and falls. His wife tells you that 2 weeks ago he had been fine, but he has been becoming progressively more confused over this period. He suffers from essential hypertension, for which he takes amlodipine, but is otherwise well. You request baseline bloods, which reveal Hb 13.5, WCC 8.96, Plts 345, Na 136, K 4.8, urea 16, creatinine 224, CRP < 5.

1. Generally, how can acute kidney injury be subclassified? **(1)**
2. Give two causes of each. **(3)**
3. Other than blood tests, give two other investigations you would request. **(2)**
4. Name two potentially life-threatening complications of acute kidney injury. **(2)**
5. Give two indications for dialysis in a patient with acute kidney injury. **(2)**

**5** An 83-year-old man is admitted to hospital via A&E. He had been found by his son on the floor in his kitchen. He is confused and unable to give any history to indicate how he fell and how long he had been on the floor. His son became concerned when he wasn't answering the phone. The last time someone had spoken to him was 24 hours prior to admission. He has a past medical history of hypertension, type 2 diabetes, BPH and osteoarthritis. His regular medications are:

- lisinopril 20 mg OD
- amlodipine 5 mg OD
- metformin 1 g BD
- gliclazide 80 mg OD.

Admission bloods are as follows: Hb 12.6, WCC 8.75, Neut 6.98, Na 135, K 5.3, urea 19.6, creatinine 352. The nurse in A&E said his urine was brown, and tested positive for blood.

1. Given the above history, what is the most likely cause of his acute kidney injury? **(1)**
2. By what mechanism does this cause acute kidney injury? **(1)**
3. What blood test would you expect to be raised in the condition you gave in 1? **(1)**
4. What urine test would you request to confirm the diagnosis? **(1)**
5. What may be seen on urine microscopy? **(1)**
6. Which medications would you hold on admission and why? **(2)**
7. Other than prolonged immobility, give three causes of this condition. **(3)**

**Q6** A 42-year-old woman has been visiting her GP regularly for 2 weeks complaining of low-grade fever, malaise and general fatigue. She had previously been fit and well. Her GP sent off routine bloods, and she has been called into hospital by the out-of-hours GP service due to the following U&Es: Na⁺ 143, K⁺ 7.4, urea 24.3, creatinine 294. These have been repeated on admission: Na⁺ 145, K⁺ 7.1, urea 23.9, creatinine 301.

1. The staff nurse hands you an ECG. Give three changes you will be looking for. **(3)**
2. You believe the ECG shows subtle changes associated with hyperkalaemia. How will you treat this initially? **(3)**
3. Her ECG changes resolve. She is afebrile, not tachycardic and is normotensive. On examination, her heart sounds are normal, chest is clear, abdomen soft, non-tender throughout, she has no neurology, no skin changes and no joint inflammation. Her urine dip reveals 2+ blood and 3+ protein. You suspect she may have a rapidly progressive glomerulonephritis. What blood tests should be requested urgently? **(2)**
4. What medication should be started immediately? **(1)**
5. The renal team review and suspect Wegener's granulomatosis. What further investigation may they request to confirm the diagnosis? **(1)**

**Q7** Mr A, a 48-year-old man, presents with a 3-week history of leg swelling that is worse when standing and walking, but resolved by lying flat. He says he has been otherwise well, has no leg pain, no shortness of breath and no chest pain. His urine dip reveals microscopic haematuria (2+) and proteinuria (3+).

1. Define nephrotic syndrome. **(1)**
2. What is the commonest cause of the nephrotic syndrome in: (a) children; (b) adults? **(2)**
3. What investigation will give a definitive diagnosis? **(1)**
4. Give two complications of nephrotic syndrome. **(2)**
5. Give one measure you would take to manage each of the above answers. **(2)**
6. Give two pieces of dietary advice you would give to a patient with nephrotic syndrome. **(2)**

**8** Mrs V is a 78-year-old lady who had visited her GP complaining of nausea and malaise for the past month. She had bloods taken at the practice this morning, and has been called by the out-of-hours GP service, who have arranged an acute medical admission due to hyponatraemia. Her bloods are repeated on admission, which reveal: Hb 12.6, WCC 7.32, Plts 255, Na 118, K 4.5, urea 5.3, creatinine 76, glucose 6.1

1. Calculate her serum osmolality. **(1)**
2. Is this high, normal or low? **(1)**
3. In order to determine the cause of hyponatraemia, you need to establish Mrs V's volume status. Give three clinical observations and investigations you could use to determine this. **(3)**
4. What is the risk of correcting chronic hyponatraemia too quickly? **(1)**
5. Where is ADH (vasopressin) secreted? **(1)**
6. How does ADH increase water reabsorption? **(1)**
7. You determine that she is euvolaemic. Her urine osmolality is 593 mmol/kg and urinary sodium is 52. What is your diagnosis? **(1)**
8. Name a drug that may be used to treat this condition. **(1)**

**9** An 18-year-old lady visits her GP complaining of dysuria and urinary frequency. On examination, she is afebrile, haemodynamically stable and her abdomen is soft, non-tender. You suspect she has cystitis.

1. Which organism is most commonly responsible for infections of the urinary tract? **(1)**
2. Give four risk factors for urinary tract infections. **(2)**
3. You perform a dipstick test on her urine. Positive results to which two reagents indicate the presence of an infection? **(2)**
4. Her urine dip suggests the presence of infection. Which antibiotic would you prescribe and for how many days? **(2)**
5. The patient states that she often suffers with UTIs and asks whether there is anything she can do to prevent them occurring. Give her three pieces of advice. **(3)**

**Q10** A 22-year-old lady has been referred by her GP with fever and severe right-sided loin pain. Her urine dip is positive for leucocytes and nitrites, and her GP suspects acute pyelonephritis. You are asked to clerk the patient.

1. Briefly outline four points of your clerking. **(4)**
2. List four investigations you would request. **(2)**

Following your assessment and analysis of investigation results, you also suspect pyelonephritis. She is treated with IV co-amoxiclav. Soon after starting antibiotics, she becomes more unwell, and you are concerned she may be having an anaphylactic reaction and treat her with hydrocortisone, chlorpheniramine and adrenaline.

3. Name two signs/symptoms you may find on assessment of her:
   (a) airway; (b) breathing; (c) circulation. **(3)**
4. Which route will you give the adrenaline, what concentration and how much? **(1)**

**Q11** An 18-year-old man presented to his GP with frequent episodes of macroscopic haematuria. He is referred to a consultant nephrologist, who suspects IgA nephropathy. His renal function is preserved, proteinuria is not in the nephrotic range and he is normotensive. He has arranged for a renal biopsy to confirm the diagnosis. You are called to speak to the patient prior to his biopsy. He is nervous and asking why the biopsy is necessary. He would also like information on the associated risks.

1. What is the benefit of renal biopsy in this case? **(1)**
2. Give two contraindications to renal biopsy. **(2)**
3. Name three complications of renal biopsy. **(3)**
4. Give one histological finding in a patient with IgA nephropathy. **(1)**

IgA nephropathy has an association with Henoch–Schönlein purpura (HSP), which commonly causes a purpuric rash on the extensor surfaces of the legs.

5. Give three other causes of a purpuric rash. **(3)**

# Rheumatology

**Q1** A 39-year-old lady is seen in the outpatient rheumatology clinic. She presents with worsening joint pains over the past few months, affecting both hands, wrists and occasionally her knees. The symptoms tend to be worse after she has woken up. A diagnosis of rheumatoid arthritis is made and a number of investigations requested.

1. Name an immunological investigation that may be requested. **(1)**
2. Give three findings you may expect to find in her hands. **(3)**
3. Give three abnormalities that may be seen on X-ray of her hands. **(3)**
4. Give four extra-articular features of rheumatoid arthritis. **(2)**
5. Further examination reveals a palpable spleen, and blood test results include a neutrophil count of 1.10. What is your revised diagnosis? **(1)**

**Q2** A 42-year-old lady presents to her GP with a 6-week history of severe pain, stiffness and swelling in the joints of her hands. Her mother was diagnosed with rheumatoid arthritis many years ago, and she suspects this is what she has. Examination of her hands reveals erythema and swelling over the interphalangeal joints bilaterally and at the wrist joint. There are no obvious bony deformities, and passive movements at these joints reveal stiffness and pain.

1. Give three other possible causes of a polyarthritis. **(3)**
2. She is seen by a rheumatologist, who diagnoses RA. She is started on regular NSAIDs. What is their mechanism of action? **(2)**
3. She is also started on methotrexate. How is this administered and how frequently is it given? **(2)**
4. Given that she is taking regular methotrexate, what drug should she also be taking? **(1)**
5. Other than her GP and rheumatologist, give two healthcare professionals who may be involved with her care. **(2)**

**Q3** A 52-year-old man presents with a 1-day history of severe pain and swelling in his big toe. He suffers from hypertension, but is otherwise fit and well. He takes ramipril and bendroflumethiazide, which was started by his GP last week.

1. What is the most likely diagnosis? **(1)**
2. What is the most likely precipitant in this case? **(1)**
3. Give three other common precipitants of this condition. **(3)**
4. Other than analgesia, give one drug that may be given in (a) the acute setting, and (b) one that may be considered for long-term prevention. **(2)**
5. Give two possible X-ray findings. **(2)**
6. What would polarised light microscopy of the synovial fluid show? **(1)**

 **Q4** A 69-year-old lady, presents via A&E with a 2-day history of severe knee pain. Her inflammatory markers are mildly elevated, and an X-ray of the knee reveals calcification within the joint.

1. What is this X-ray finding called? **(1)**
2. What is the diagnosis? **(1)**
3. What other joints are commonly affected? **(2)**
4. Give two risk factors for this condition. **(2)**
5. What further investigation would you do perform to confirm the diagnosis? **(1)**
6. What would you expect to find from the above? **(1)**
7. Give two other possible causes of an acute monoarthritis. **(2)**

 **Q5** A 68-year-old male, who is a retired carpenter, is referred to orthopaedics by his GP with long-standing knee pain. His GP suspects that osteoarthritis is the most likely cause of his symptoms, and he has been managing him with simple analgesia in the community.

1. Give four signs that may be present on examination of the knee. **(4)**
2. An X-ray of the knee is taken. Give four changes that may be present. **(2)**
3. Give four possible treatment options. **(4)**

Q6 A 36-year-old lady was diagnosed with systemic lupus erythematosis (SLE) 5 years ago. She has been trying for a baby with her husband for some time, but unfortunately has suffered three consecutive miscarriages.

1. Give two immunological blood tests that may be positive in this patient. **(2)**
2. Give two effects of SLE that may be seen on the skin. **(2)**
3. What is the most likely cause of her recurrent miscarriage? **(1)**
4. Give the three other features of this condition. **(3)**
5. Give two drugs that may be used to treat this condition. **(2)**

Q7 A 39-year-old lady is referred to the rheumatology clinic with weight loss, malaise and proximal muscle weakness, mainly affecting her shoulders. On examination, she does have proximal muscle weakness. Also noted is a purple discolouration of her eyelids and rough, red papules over her knuckles. It is suspected that she has dermatomyositis.

1. What is the name given to the purple discolouration of her eyelids? **(1)**
2. What is the name given to the rough, red papules over her knuckles? **(1)**
3. Name two autoantibodies associated with this condition. **(2)**

The next patient in the clinic has limited cutaneous scleroderma. One feature of this is Raynaud's phenomenon.

4. What is Raynaud's phenomenon? **(1)**
5. Give three causes of Raynaud's phenomenon, other than scleroderma. **(3)**
6. Give the four other classical features of limited cutaneous scleroderma. **(2)**

**8** A 22-year-old man presents with a 4-week history of progressively worsening lower back pain, radiating towards his buttocks and hips. He has associated stiffness in the lower back that appears to be worse when he wakes up, and he finds exercising helps to reduce this. You suspect ankylosing spondylitis.

1. Give two other seronegative spondyloarthropathies. **(2)**
2. Which antigen tends to be positive in the majority of patients with these conditions? **(1)**
3. Describe the classical radiographic changes seen in ankylosing spondylitis? **(2)**
4. Give two medical options for management of ankylosing spondylitis. **(2)**

Four months later, the same patient visits his GP, with severe pain and photophobia in his right eye. On examination, his visual acuity is 6/6 in his left eye and 6/24 in his right eye.

5. What diagnosis must be excluded? **(1)**
6. As part of your assessment, you also listen to his heart and lungs. What added sounds may you hear? **(2)**

**9** A 42-year-old man with known plaque psoriasis also has psoriatic arthritis.

1. Other than chronic plaque psoriasis, name two other forms of psoriasis. **(2)**
2. Give two sites that the skin lesions of chronic plaque psoriasis commonly affect. **(1)**
3. Some patients with psoriatic arthritis develop periarticular osteolysis and shortnening of the bones. What is this form of psoriatic arthritis called? **(1)**

Psoriatic arthritis is a seronegative arthritis, as are reactive arthritis and Reiter's syndrome.

4. Name three organisms that may trigger reactive arthritis. **(3)**
5. What are the three features of Reiter's syndrome? **(3)**

**Q10** A 34-year-old lady is regularly seen by a rheumatologist and also by the renal clinic for management of Wegener's granulomatosis, a small-vessel vasculitis. This was diagnosed following a renal biopsy which revealed characteristic changes, and an autoimmune screen in keeping with this.

1. Name one other ANCA +ve small-vessel vasculitis, and one ANCA –ve small-vessel vasculitis. **(2)**
2. Name one large-vessel vasculitis and one medium-vessel vasculitis. **(2)**
3. Name two systemic conditions in which vasculitis is a feature of the disease. **(2)**

Wegener's granulomatosis is an important cause of mononeuritis multiplex, a term used to describe inflammation or damage to ≥ 2 peripheral nerves.

4. Name four other causes of mononeuritis multiplex. **(4)**

# Endocrinology

Q1  A 49-year-old gentleman and his wife come to you in the GP practice, with his wife stating that he is having trouble taking his wedding ring off and he has noticed that he has had to buy larger shoes over the last 2 years or so. His wife also states that he is becoming very clumsy around the house and is constantly bumping into things. You suspect acromegaly.

1. What is acromegaly? **(1)**
2. State six signs or symptoms you might look for on questioning and examination of this man. **(3)**
3. How do you account for his wife's statement? **(1)**
4. What serum blood test do you want to perform to screen for acromegaly? **(1)**
5. Explain how an oral glucose tolerance test (OGTT) can aid diagnosis. **(1)**

Testing confirms acromegaly.
6. What other endocrinological disorder would you now screen for? Explain your answer. **(1)**
7. In general terms, what is the main cause of death in these patients? **(1)**
8. What surgery is performed in the hope of curing these patients? **(1)**

Q2 A 68-year-old lady comes to see you in the GP surgery. She complains of feeling tired, is gaining weight and complaining of feeling constantly cold in the house. She has some cardiovascular disease, for which is taking amiodarone, aspirin and simvastatin. She also suffers with asthma, which is well controlled on salbutamol and beclomethasone. In the past, she had pharyngeal cancer, which was treated with radiotherapy successfully. You suspect hypothyroidism.

1. From her past medical history, name two possible causes of the hypothyroidism. **(1)**
2. Name four other signs you may find on examination. **(2)**
3. Name two possible causes of hypothyroidism in this patient, other than the two you have suggested in 1. **(2)**

You decide to order thyroid function tests and a full blood count.

4. What might the full blood count show? **(1)**
5. With the use of 'high', 'low' or 'normal', what will the level of TSH and $T_4$ be in a patient with primary hypothyroidism? **(1)**
6. How would you treat this patient medically? **(1)**
7. The patient then admits to noticing some 'very white patches' on the back of both her hands. What could this represent? **(1)**
8. What anatomical structure represents the site at which the thyroid gland originated before embryological descent? **(1)**

Q3 A 62-year-old lady comes to your GP practice complaining of weight loss despite 'eating like a horse', and she has noticed a fine tremor in her hands. She is also frustrated with her husband putting the heating on, as she states that she is always feels very warm, even when her husband says he is cold. You suspect hyperthroidism.

1. What is Graves' disease? **(1)**
2. Name three signs you might look for on examination of the above condition. **(3)**
3. What do you expect her thyroid function tests to show? **(1)**
4. What drug class could be used to control her tremor? **(1)**
5. Name two drugs that could be used to treat this patient long-term, to 'block the thyroid'. **(2)**
6. Name two signs on examination that are specific for Graves' disease (you may have already mentioned them in 2). **(2)**

**Q4** A 25-year-old lady comes to you with symptoms of excessive thirst, weight loss and increase in urine production. Her urine dipstick is negative for glucose.

1. What is the likely diagnosis? **(1)**
2. Where is ADH secreted from? **(1)**
3. With the use of 'low', 'high' and 'normal', what do you expect her urine osmolality and plasma osmolality to be? **(2)**
4. What's the difference between the nephrogenic and cranial types of this condition? **(2)**
5. Explain how the water deprivation test is used to diagnose the condition. **(2)**
6. Name the drug used to treat the cranial type of this condition. **(1)**

On further questioning, she recently gave birth to her son, but after delivery suffered a massive post-partum haemorrhage.

7. With this information, what do you think the cause of her condition might be? **(1)**

**Q5** A teenage boy is rushed into A&E, with his parents looking very concerned. They were unable to fully rouse him from bed this morning; he is unresponsive. He is a known diabetic.

1. What would be your first bedside test? **(1)**
2. Give two ways of raising the glucose level in this patient. **(2)**
3. What do you think is the likely cause of the hypoglycaemia? **(1)**
4. Name two symptoms of neuroglycopenia other than coma. **(2)**
5. What can repeated episodes of hypoglycaemia lead to? **(1)**
6. What advice would you give to the patient and his family regarding prevention of future episodes? **(2)**
7. Name a cause of hypoglycaemia in non-diabetic patients. **(1)**

**Q6** A 54-year-old obese gentleman comes to see you in the GP practice, complaining of a persistent fungal infection of the glans of his penis. On further questioning, he complains of tiredness and visual blurring over the past 3 months, and has noticed that he is passing large volumes of urine.

1. What is the underlying diagnosis? **(1)**
2. Explain the oral glucose tolerance test. **(3)**
3. Name two macrovascular and two microvascular complications of the condition you have identified in 1. **(2)**
4. Name three different agents that could be used to treat this gentleman's underlying condition. **(3)**
5. What advice would you give this gentleman? **(1)**

**Q7** A 17-year-old girl with no past medical history is bought into A&E resus with persistent vomiting, hyperventilation and confusion. Her blood glucose is 28 mmol/L. Your consultant tells you this is likely diabetic ketoacidosis.

1. How do you confirm the diagnosis on bedside testing? **(1)**
2. Name two venous blood tests you would perform now. **(2)**

An arterial blood gas is performed, giving:
pH 7.11
$PO_2$ 13.8 kPa
$PCO_2$ 2.7 kPa
BE −7.3
$HCO_3$ 18.9 mmol/L.

3. What is your interpretation of this blood gas? **(1)**
4. What management would you initiate? **(3)**
5. Explain the pathophysiology of diabetic ketoacidosis? **(3)**

**8** A 40-year-old man presents to you complaining of feeling tired all the time and loss of appetite. He has a past medical history of vitiligo. Examination is unremarkable except some slight tanning of the skin and buccal pigmentation.

1. In light of the history and examination findings, what do you suspect the diagnosis and pathogenesis is? **(2)**
2. Name two tests you would like to perform to aid diagnosis? **(2)**
3. With use of 'low', 'high' and 'normal', what would you expect his serum sodium and potassium to be classically? **(2)**
4. Apart from glucocorticoids, what other drug class will you prescribe this man? **(1)**
5. What advice would have to be given this man after prescribing him glucocorticoids? **(3)**

**9** A 28-year-old girl presents to you because she has become amenorrhoeic. You do a serum prolactin that comes back as 2850 mU/L.

1. What is the commonest cause of pathological hyperprolactinaemia? **(1)**
2. Name three other signs or symptoms she may have. **(3)**
3. What imaging test will you request? **(1)**
4. Why will you also order visual field testing? Explain your answer. **(2)**

Testing confirms prolactinoma. You advise the patient that she requires surgery; however, she states she does not want surgery and is willing for any other form of treatment.

5. Name a drug that can be used to treat her and its mechanism of action. **(2)**
6. What other treatment option is available to her? **(1)**

**Q10** A 60-year-old lady comes to you complaining of tiredness and abdominal pain over the last few months. She has no past medical history of note. On routine blood testing, her correct calcium is 3.08 mmol/L.
  1. Name three other symptoms or signs she may have? **(3)**
  2. What blood test would you now order? **(1)**

Primary hyperparathyroidism is confirmed.
  3. With the use of 'low', 'high' or 'normal', what would you expect the phosphate level to be? **(1)**
  4. What imaging tests would you order? **(2)**
  5. Name two specific complications of surgical resection of parathyroid adenoma. **(2)**
  6. What is the relationship between vitamin D and calcium? **(1)**

**Q11** A 69-year-old obese gentleman with long-standing type 2 diabetes presents to you with a diminished sensation in his hands and feet. You diagnose a symmetrical polyneuropathy secondary to his poorly controlled diabetes.
  1. What is the common term used to describe the distribution of this gentleman's diminished sensation? **(1)**
  2. On examination, in this particular neuropathy, what is the first type of sense to diminish? **(1)**
  3. Apart from blunted sensation, what else might you find on examination of this man's feet? **(2)**
  4. Name two other types of neuropathy that can occur in diabetic patients? **(2)**
  5. What is key in his management to preventing progression of his polyneuropthy? **(1)**
  6. In light of finding a neuropathy which is a microvascular complication of diabetes, what two other areas of the body must now be investigated? **(2)**

He comes back some months later with intractable vomiting.
  7. In light of his previous history, how do you explain the vomiting? **(1)**

# Haematology

Q1 Daniel, a 21-year-old man, presents to you complaining of feeling an enlarged lump in his neck for the past 6 weeks. You examine it and find it to be 3 cm by 2 cm, painless on palpation and with a 'rubbery' feel to it. You suspect lymphoma.
  1. List three symptoms he may also complain of. **(3)**
  2. Name two signs you will look for on examination. **(2)**

The biopsy shows the presence of a binucleated cell. The haematologist states it is Hodgkin's lymphoma.
  3. What is the name of this cell that suggests Hodgkin's lymphoma? **(1)**
  4. State two staging investigations. **(2)**
  5. What staging system is classically used for Hodgkin's lymphoma? **(1)**

Whilst being investigated, Daniel presents to A&E with dyspnoea, swelling of the face and congested veins in his neck and chest.
  6. What has happened? **(1)**

**Q2** A 44-year-old Afro-Caribbean lady comes to see you in the GP practice with menorrhagia. You decide to do a full blood count, the results of which are:

Hb 7.8 g/dL
MCV 75 fL
Platelets 398 × 10⁹/L
WCC 8.8 × 10⁹/L

1. Describe the above full blood count. **(2)**
2. Name three signs the patient may have on examination. **(3)**

You decide she is most likely iron deficient secondary to the heavy bleeding.

3. Name one other cause of iron-deficiency anaemia. **(1)**
4. Name two more specific signs that may be present on examining somebody with chronic iron-deficiency anaemia. **(2)**

One part of your management plan includes prescribing ferrous sulphate. She asks if there are any common side effects to the drug.

5. Name two common side effects of ferrous sulphate. **(2)**

**Q3** A 33-year-old known sickle-cell patient comes into the walk-in haematology clinic complaining of acute severe leg pain. He has no history of trauma and is otherwise fit and well, however over the past week he has been treated for an upper respiratory tract infection. You diagnose sickle-cell crisis.

1. As he is a long-term patient with severe sickle-cell disease, what would you expect him to have in his drug history? Name two drugs. **(2)**
2. Other than infection, name two factors that can bring on a sickle-cell crisis? **(2)**
3. State three general points in managing this patient. **(3)**
4. What is the pattern of inheritance of sickle-cell disease? **(1)**
5. With the above answer in mind, what is the likelihood of his children having sickle-cell trait if his partner has normal chromosomes? **(1)**
6. Why does sickle-cell disease not usually clinically manifest until roughly 6 months of age? **(1)**

**4** A 70-year-old man comes to see you in the GP practice with lower backache that has been going on for 3 months. After referring him for some X-rays of the spine and hips, they show spinal crush fracture and punched-out lesions in the pelvis. You are worried that this is multiple myeloma.

1. What is multiple myeloma? **(1)**
2. What is the commonest immunoglobulin expressed as part of the disease? **(1)**
3. State two other common symptoms a patient with multiple myeloma may complain of. **(2)**
4. State three investigations you would perform except X-rays. **(3)**
5. Why are these patients prone to bacterial infections? **(3)**
6. State four acute complications of myeloma. **(2)**

**5** A 40-year-old lady comes to see you complaining of general tiredness and a feeling of fullness in the abdomen that have come on over the past 6 months. You examine her, and find she looks pale and has splenomegaly measuring five fingers' breadth under the costal margin. You suspect chronic leukaemia.

1. Name two causes for splenomegaly other than leukaemia. **(2)**
2. What would you expect the WCC to be on her full blood count if this is chronic leukaemia – low, normal or high? **(1)**

A blood film is ordered, which is highly suggestive of chronic leukaemia.

3. In general terms, how could you differentiate (on a blood film) between acute leukaemia and chronic leukaemia? **(2)**

A bone marrow aspirate is performed by the haematologist at the local hospital that shows (on cytogenetic testing) a characteristic translocation of chronic myeloid leukaemia (CML) between chromosomes 9 and 22.

4. What is the name given to this characteristic abnormal chromosome? **(1)**
5. Name the breakthrough drug used to treat CML, its mechanism of action and the route in which it is taken. **(3)**

Six months later, a repeat bone marrow aspirate is done which still shows the presence of 95% of cells having the same genetic abnormality.

6. What would be an appropriate next step in treatment? **(1)**

Q6 A 55-year-old gentleman is referred urgently to the haematology clinic after suffering from breathlessness and widespread petechiae which have rapidly worsened over a 7-day period. He also complains of bone pain in his legs. A WCC of 98 × 10⁹/L on his FBC is also on the referral letter. You are worried about a possible haematological malignancy.

1.  Bone marrow failure will give what three findings on full blood count? **(3)**
2.  How do you account for his bone pain? **(1)**
3.  What is the next immediate investigation you would order? **(1)**

A bone marrow aspirate shows the dominating presence of blast cells of the myeloid lineage.

4.  What is the diagnosis? **(2)**

The haematology team manages him. They plan to start chemotherapy and aim for stem cell transplantation.

5.  What supportive treatment will he need? **(3)**

**7** A 19-year-old male is brought into A&E after a motorcycle injury in which he fractured his pelvis and both femurs. After the acute care team stabilise him, they ask you to perform a full blood count. The Hb comes back as 5.9 g/dL.

1. Below what value of haemoglobin should a blood transfusion take place, regardless of symptoms? **(1)**
2. Name two signs that may be present specific to his haemoglobin level? **(2)**

You decide to transfuse 4 units. Fifteen minutes into the first bag of blood being transfused, a nurse comes to you urgently to say the patient's temperature has increased to 38.4°C and his blood pressure has dropped to 79/47 mmHg.

3. Name one differential diagnosis of the type of transfusion reaction occurring? **(1)**
4. What is your first management step? **(1)**

You notice oozing from the cannula site and the puncture wound from a failed cannula attempt earlier on.

5. What haematological state has occurred secondary to the transfusion reaction? **(1)**
6. Name one other type of 'early' (within 24 hours) transfusion complication (other than the one you have mentioned in 3) and one 'late' (after 24 hours) transfusion complication. **(2)**
7. What is the definition of a massive blood transfusion? **(2)**

**8** Alice is a 68-year-old lady with a past medical history of vitiligo and Addison's disease. She comes to see you, saying she has been feeling lethargic over the past few months. You take a full blood count, which reveals a macrocytic anaemia.

1. How can macrocytic anaemia be classified into two categories? Name two causes in each category of macrocytic anaemia. **(6)**
2. What test is required to distinguish the two categories? **(1)**
3. What do you think might be the cause in Alice's case? **(1)**
4. Name a test you could use to help confirm your suspicions. **(1)**
5. How will you treat Alice? **(1)**

Q9 A worried Cypriot mother comes to see you with her 2-year-old son, complaining that he has stunted growth and she has found he is much less active than he was 6 months ago. Before you refer on to a paediatrician, you decide to do a full blood count, the results of which are:

Hb 6 g/dL

MCV 63 fL

MCH 25 Hb/cell (normal range 31–38)

You suspect thalassaemia major.
1. Describe the above full blood count. **(3)**
2. What signs would you look for on examination? Name two. **(2)**

Serum electrophoresis confirms beta-thalassaemia major.
3. What is the common name given to beta-thalassaemia major? **(1)**
4. What are the two main treatments for beta-thalassaemia major? **(2)**
5. What will you offer the mother as a part of your management? **(1)**
6. Why does thalassaemia major never usually present in the first 6 months of life? **(1)**

Q10 A mother brings her young son into the A&E department, complaining that her son has severe pain in his shin area after gently knocking it whilst playing football in the garden. He has pain in the shin area on passive movement of the ankle, he is unable to move his ankle himself and the lower leg looks pale as well as having decreased sensation. He has known severe haemophilia A and you also notice that he has chronic joint deformity of both knees and his right elbow.
1. What is being described in the acute presentation and what is the usual management of this? **(2)**
2. How do you account for the joint deformities? **(1)**
3. How is haemophilia A inherited? **(2)**
4. Which clotting factor is deficient in haemophilia A? **(1)**
5. With the use of 'decreased', 'normal' and 'prolonged', what would you expect to see on clotting studies of his INR and APTT? **(2)**
6. Name a treatment that can be given to these patients to improve their clotting factor deficiency. **(1)**
7. How would you account for a lady being diagnosed with haemophilia A at the age of 70? **(1)**

# Gastroenterology

**Q1** Richard, aged 25, comes to see you with a 3-month history of diarrhoea, abdominal pain and weight loss.

1. List four differential diagnoses for chronic diarrhoea in this age group. **(2)**
2. Name a basic test and an invasive test that could help with diagnosis. **(2)**
3. Richard undergoes a biopsy, which states in its conclusion, 'Features suggestive of Crohn's disease'. List two histological features of Crohn's disease. **(2)**
4. Contrast Crohn's disease and ulcerative colitis in the following domains: endoscopic appearance and distribution. **(3)**
5. List two extraintestinal features of Crohn's disease. **(2)**
6. Supportive therapy, oral prednisolone or IV hydrocortisone is the mainstay of medical treatment in acute flare-ups. However, steroid-sparing agents such as azathioprine and methotrexate are frequently used. Why are steroid-sparing agents useful? **(1)**
7. List two complications from long-term Crohn's disease. **(2)**
8. Infliximab is a monoclonal antibody that can reduce Crohn's disease activity. How does it work? **(1)**

Q2  Fred, aged 52, is brought into A&E following an episode of vomiting a
large quantity of blood.

1. List four causes of upper GI bleeding. **(2)**
2. A drug history in Fred's case is important. What three medications
   can contribute to an upper GI bleed? **(2)**
3. What may be gained from rectal examination in Fred's case? **(1)**
4. After initial fluid resuscitation, his blood investigations are back
   from the lab. Explain the following results: haemoglobin 13.0,
   urea 14.5, creatinine 67. **(2)**
5. What diagnostic investigation is indicated? **(1)**
6. What class of medication can be given? **(1)**
7. On urgent examination, a diagnosis of oesophageal varices is
   made. What disease is this commonly associated with? **(1)**
8. What is the mechanism by which your answer to 7 leads to
   oesophageal varices? **(1)**
9. Name a site of portosystemic anastomoses and the symptom it
   would cause. **(2)**
10. Name an endoscopic treatment of oesophageal varices. **(1)**

Q3 Neil, aged 42, comes to see you, complaining of a burning pain in the epigastric region when he eats and in the evening. You suspect Neil has peptic ulcer disease.

1. Name two differential diagnoses for dyspepsia other than peptic ulcer disease. **(2)**
2. Name two symptoms that would alert you to the possibility of upper GI malignancy. **(2)**
3. List two risk factors for peptic ulcer disease. **(2)**
4. You decide to perform a urease breath test for *H. pylori*. Explain the basis of this test. **(2)**
5. It transpires that Neil has *H. pylori* in his stomach. What is the basis for *H. pylori* eradication? **(2)**
6. Many months later, Neil presents to A&E with severe upper abdominal pain. What radiological investigation would you use to look for possible perforation? **(1)**
7. What sign would you be looking for in the investigation you listed in 6? **(1)**
8. Once perforation has been ruled out, what invasive investigation could aid diagnosis? **(1)**
9. Abnormally high gastrin levels are associated with extensive and atypical ulceration. What is the name of the condition that causes this? **(2)**

Q4 Maria, a 47-year-old, comes to see you regarding her heartburn and acid regurgitation. She says it is getting worse, despite using over-the-counter antacids.

1. What is the definition of gastro-oesphageal reflux disease (GORD)? **(1)**
2. List two exacerbating factors of GORD. **(2)**
3. Maria has also been suffering from wheeze at night-time, but has no history of asthma. What could be causing wheeze? **(1)**
4. What lifestyle changes could you offer? **(2)**
5. You try her with a course of lansoprazole 30 mg, which initially works. However, 6 months later, she comes back to see you with the same symptoms, plus difficulty swallowing. Name two causes of dysphagia in this case. **(2)**
6. You send Maria for urgent upper GI endoscopy, where biopsies are taken. The histology report is as follows: 'Microscopy shows oesophageal metaplasia suggestive of Barrett's oesophagus'. Explain the term 'oesophageal metaplasia' and its cause. **(2)**
7. What is the gold-standard test for proving reflux? **(1)**
8. Maria sees a specialist who suggests surgical treatment with a Nissen fundoplication, where the fundus is wrapped around the abdominal oesophagus. How may this help reflux? **(1)**
9. Name a possible side effect specific to fundoplication. **(1)**

**Q5**  Janine, aged 62, is admitted from A&E with new-onset jaundice.

1. Give one example for each of the following causes of jaundice: prehepatic, intrahepatic/hepatocellular, cholestatic/obstructive. **(3)**
2. What is bilirubin a breakdown product of? **(1)**
3. Janine also complains of dark urine and pale stools. Which of the causes listed in 1 are her symptoms likely to be due to? **(1)**
4. Why does conjugated bilirubin appear in the urine and unconjugated bilirubin doesn't? **(1)**
5. What non-invasive radiological investigation is indicated in this case? **(1)**
6. The above investigation showed an 8-mm dilated CBD and a pancreatic mass. What invasive procedure could be diagnostic and therapeutic? **(1)**
7. Cytology obtained from the above procedure is suggestive of pancreatic carcinoma. What is the commonest histological type of pancreatic carcinoma? **(1)**
8. Name two other symptoms and signs of pancreatic cancer. **(2)**
9. What tumour marker can be used to monitor response to pancreatic cancer treatment? **(1)**
10. Janine has ongoing jaundice. Name a complication of persistent jaundice. **(1)**

**Q6**  Daryl, aged 31, presents to the emergency department with a 2-month history of gradual-onset jaundice, and feeling generally unwell with a fever. His blood is sent for liver function tests. The results are as follows: bilirubin 102, ALT 940, AST 847, ALP 204.

1. What pattern of liver damage do these LFTs reflect? **(1)**
2. What are the routes of spread of hepatitis A and hepatitis B? **(2)**
3. Daryl tests positive for HBsAg. List two 'at-risk groups' for hepatitis B. **(2)**
4. What does having antibodies to hepatitis B core antigen (anti-HBC) in the serum signify? **(1)**
5. Name two long-term complications of hepatitis B. **(2)**
6. A healthcare worker takes some repeat bloods from Daryl and sustains a needle-stick injury. What should the healthcare worker do now? **(1)**
7. Name two viruses that Daryl may be co-infected with. **(2)**

**Q7** Ted, aged 46, is admitted to the medical admissions unit with confusion. He is known to have liver cirrhosis.

1. What is the commonest cause of liver cirrhosis in the UK? **(1)**
2. Name an example of both a hereditary cause of cirrhosis and an acquired cause of cirrhosis. **(2)**
3. Name two signs of chronic liver disease that you may find on examination. **(2)**
4. Name two investigations to test the synthetic function of the liver. **(2)**
5. Name two complications of cirrhosis. **(2)**
6. Ted has a tense abdomen with shifting dullness. How would you treat Ted's ascites? **(2)**
7. Ascitic fluid is sent to the pathology lab. Name two investigations you should order. **(2)**
8. Ted is thought to have severe hepatic encephalopathy. Sedatives are avoided and he is given lactulose. What is the rationale for using lactulose? **(1)**
9. What is the only definitive treatment for liver cirrhosis? **(1)**

**Q8** Lucy, aged 24, comes to see you in the GP surgery with a history of chronic abdominal pain. She has lost 10 kg unintentionally in the last 3 months. She is worried about coeliac disease.

1. List two other causes of GI malabsorption. **(2)**
2. How else might coeliac disease present? Give two examples. **(2)**
3. What is the aetiology of coeliac disease? **(1)**
4. What is the commonest source of gluten? **(1)**
5. You send Lucy for tissue anti-endomysial serology, an IgA antibody. Name another blood test you could send her for. **(1)**
6. In severe malabsorption from coeliac disease, why may anti-endomysial antibodies be negative? **(1)**
7. Lucy is sent for upper GI endoscopy, where duodenal biopsies are taken. Name a feature of coeliac disease on histology. **(1)**
8. What is the treatment of coeliac disease? **(1)**
9. Name two autoimmune diseases that coeliac disease may be associated with. **(2)**
10. Name two cancers associated with coeliac disease. **(2)**

**9** Sally, aged 39, comes to see you with a long-term history of abdominal pain and alternating constipation and diarrhoea.

1. Give an example of the following causes of constipation: drug-induced, mechanical and lifestyle. **(3)**
2. Name two other symptoms of irritable bowel syndrome (IBS). **(2)**
3. When considering IBS as a diagnosis, organic disease should be ruled out. Why are the following tests performed: full blood count, thyroid function tests and sigmoidoscopy? **(3)**
4. Name a psychological disorder associated with IBS. **(1)**
5. Many months later, Sally comes to see you again with weight loss, fatigue and increasing abdominal pain. Further blood testing reveals new iron-deficiency anaemia. What invasive investigation should you refer her for? Explain your answer. **(2)**
6. Name two predisposing factors to colonic carcinoma. **(2)**
7. Name a site to where colorectal cancer may metastasise. **(1)**

**10** Tristan, aged 22, has come to the emergency department with a day-long history of profuse watery diarrhoea and vomiting. You think he may have gastroenteritis.

1. Name two bacteria that may cause acute diarrhoea. **(2)**
2. Name a viral cause of gastroenteritis. **(1)**
3. Name three symptomatic treatments you can give. **(3)**
4. Tristan was recently treated with ciprofloxacin for a sexually transmitted infection. What may Tristan be at risk of? **(1)**
5. What medications can be used to treat your answer above? **(2)**
6. What infection-control measures should be used when treating acute diarrhoea? **(2)**

# Neurology

Q1  A 42-year-old man attends A&E complaining of the worst headache he
has ever experienced. It came on suddenly 1 hour ago and affects the
occipital region. He also complains of neck stiffness. He has been feeling well over this week and last saw his GP 1 year ago after having the
coryzal symptoms. You suspect a subarachnoid haemorrhage (SAH).

1. Is this an arterial or venous intracranial haemorrhage? **(1)**
2. What is the type of aneurysm that commonly causes SAH? **(1)**
3. Name a condition associated with this type of aneurysm. **(1)**
4. Name four symptoms or signs the may patient experience other
   than a headache? **(2)**
5. What is Kernig's sign and what does it demonstrate? **(2)**
6. What imaging would you request and what would it classically
   show you? **(2)**
7. What further test would you perform if the imaging does not
   demonstrate any abnormality and what would you ask the
   laboratory to analyse for? **(2)**

**2** An 18-year-old man attends A&E after being hit in the temple with a cricket bat in a fight that broke out in his town centre. He initially lost consciousness at the scene, but after coming round, walked home, where his mother found him confused. On arrival, he opens his eyes to voice, withdraws from painful stimulus and is confused and disorientated.

1. What is his GCS? **(1)**
2. What is the term for the period when he was awake following initial insult and when his GCS started to drop? **(1)**
3. What four bones meet at the pterion? **(half a mark each, max 2 marks)**
4. Is the bleed arterial or venous in an extradural haemorrhage? **(1)**
5. Is the bleed arterial or venous in a subdural haemorrhage? **(1)**
6. What are the differences in the shape of haematoma on CT head scan between extradural and subdural haematoma? **(1 mark each, max 2 marks)**
7. What other changes maybe identified on the CT scan? **(2)**

**3** A 75-year-old woman attends A&E after her daughter arrived at her house and found her slumped in her seat with left-sided facial droop and left-arm and left-leg weakness. She has previously had a CABG following an MI, has hypertension and has been a lifelong smoker. You suspect a stroke.

1. Name four risk factors for a stroke that have not been mentioned in the history above. **(2)**
2. What is the difference between a stroke and a TIA? **(1)**
3. What is the term for the left-sided weakness in this patient? **(1)**
4. Give two other signs that may accompany this weakness in a patient suffering a cerebral hemisphere infarct? **(2)**
5. What is the commonest cause of cerebral infarct and what surgical technique can be considered? **(2)**
6. An ischaemic stroke was found on CT scanning, and antiplatelet management started. Apart from medical treatment, what else should be considered in managing this patient? **(2)**

**4** A 25-year-old male attends A&E, having had a 2-minute seizure at home. It is the second time this has happened; his mother was present and witnessed his arms and legs shaking. He was unresponsive during the episode and was drowsy following it. He has been bought in by ambulance staff, who have established IV access. He has returned to GCS 15.

1. What is epilepsy? **(1)**
2. What is an 'aura'? **(1)**
3. What is Todd's palsy? **(1)**
4. What type of epilepsy is being described here? **(1)**
5. Name two other types of seizures and give a brief description. **(2)**
6. Give two metabolic causes of seizures. **(2)**

The patient starts to fit on you while you are assessing him in the department. You are concerned that he is not maintaining his airway.

7. What airway adjunct could you use? **(1)**
8. What other immediate steps would you take in managing this patient? **(2)**

**5** A 50-year-old woman attends her GP clinic complaining that she has noticed she has become clumsy and feels that her vision is not 'as wide' as it used to be. You perform a full cranial nerve examination and find that her visual fields are limited: she seems to have lost the lateral half of her vision in both eyes. She is is otherwise asymptomatic and feels well.

1. How would you describe this visual loss? **(1)**
2. What part of the visual pathway is likely to be affected? **(1)**
3. What is the likely cause for the compression and what is implied as the patient is otherwise well? **(2)**
4. Is the lateral or medial portion of the retinal field likely to be affected? **(1)**
5. The cranial nerves II, III, IV and VI are involved in vision and movement of the eye. What are the six routinely performed tests clinically to assess these cranial nerves? **(3)**
6. Damage to what two visual structures can lead to a homonymous hemianopia? **(2)**

**Q6** A 75-year-old man attends A&E after losing the ability to move both his legs. His upper limbs are unaffected. He has suffered two myocardial infarctions and has peripheral vascular disease. You decide to perform a full peripheral nerve examination and find impaired temperature and pain sensation below L1.

1. What will you test to decide whether the dorsal column is intact in the lower limbs? **(2)**
2. Does the dorsal column run anteriorly or posteriorly in the spinal cord? **(1)**
3. Where does the dorsal column decussate? **(1)**
4. What sensory modalities does the spinothalamic tract carry? **(2)**
5. What part of the spine has been affected? **(1)**
6. Given this gentleman's PMH, what would be a likely cause of his presentation? **(1)**
7. Describe the distribution of signs found for a patient with a left-sided Brown–Séquard syndrome affecting the lumbar region. **(2)**

**Q7** A 22-year-old woman goes to see her GP due to a headache. On further questioning, she is found to have fever, photophobia and neck stiffness. On examination, she is found to have a generalised petechial rash and is Kernig's sign positive. The GP is concerned about meningitis, so gives her an intramuscular antibiotic and sends her immediately to A&E. A diagnosis of bacterial meningitis is confirmed by lumbar puncture, so she is commenced on intravenous antibiotics.

1. What are the three layers of the meninges? **(3)**
2. Give the two organisms which commonly cause meningitis in this woman's age group. **(2)**
3. What is a positive Kernig's sign? **(1)**
4. What is the petechial rash found on examination indicative of? **(1)**
5. Prior to performing a lumbar puncture, why might a CT head scan be performed? **(1)**
6. What antibiotic will the GP have given her intramuscularly prior to admission to A&E? **(1)**
7. What group of antibiotics are the empirical treatment of choice for suspected bacterial meningitis once the patient is admitted to hospital? **(1)**

**Q8** A 49-year-old woman is seen by her GP with a 3-week history of numbness and tingling in the thumb, index, middle and half of the ring finger of her right hand. She reports the symptoms are worse at night. She has positive Phalen's and Tinel's tests. The GP suspects carpal tunnel syndrome.

1. Which nerve is compressed in carpal tunnel syndrome? **(1)**
2. Which muscles in the hand are supplied by this muscle? **(2)**
3. What is a positive Phalen's test? **(1)**
4. What is a positive Tinel's test? **(1)**
5. Give two risk factors for carpal tunnel syndrome. **(2)**
6. State one investigation that may be performed. **(1)**
7. What are two management options for this condition? **(2)**

**Q9** A 63-year-old man is seen by his GP, as he has developed a tremor in his right hand. On examination, he is found to have 'pill rolling' tremor at rest. The GP suspects Parkinson's disease.

1. Apart from tremor, give two clinical hallmarks of Parkinson's disease? **(2)**
2. What neurotransmitter is deficient in the substantia nigra? **(1)**
3. What is the name given to lesions seen microscopically in the brain of a patient with Parkinson's disease? **(1)**
4. When commencing levodopa, what other medication should be commenced at the same time and why? **(2)**
5. Give two complications associated with long-term levodopa treatment? **(2)**
6. Apart from levodopa, give two management options. **(2)**

Q10 A 79-year-old woman is seen by her GP due to headaches. On further questioning, her husband has noted her personality has changed recently. The GP examines her and suspects raised intracranial pressure, so sends her to A&E.

1. At what time of day is the headache in raised intracranial pressure typically worse? **(1)**
2. What may patients report exacerbates the headache? **(1)**
3. Give two clinical features other than headache which may occur due to raised intracranial pressure. **(2)**
4. Give two examples of space-occupying lesions which may be causing the raised intracranial pressure. **(2)**
5. Based on the information given above, which lobe of the brain is a space-occupying lesion likely to be affecting? **(1)**
6. What imaging should be performed in this patient in the A&E department? **(1)**
7. Give two medical managements which may be used to decrease intracranial pressure. **(2)**

# Surgery

# General surgery

**Q1** A 20-year-old man presents to A&E with abdominal pain. The pain started in the periumbilical region, but is now felt in the right iliac fossa. On examination, there is right iliac fossa tenderness with guarding and rebound tenderness. He also has a positive Rovsing's sign. A diagnosis of acute appendicitis is made.

1. Apart from abdominal pain, give two symptoms of acute appendicitis. **(2)**
2. Why is the pain first felt in the periumbilical region? **(1)**
3. Why does it then migrate to the right iliac fossa? **(1)**
4. What is Rovsing's sign? **(1)**
5. Give two differentials of appendicitis. **(2)**
6. What is the definitive treatment of appendicitis? **(1)**
7. Give two possible complications of appendicitis. **(2)**

**Q2** An 82-year-old woman is admitted to A&E with left iliac fossa pain and fever. She is diagnosed as having diverticulitis.

1. What is a diverticulum? **(1)**
2. Which section of the colon are diverticula commoner in? **(1)**
3. Define diverticulosis, diverticular disease and diverticulitis. **(3)**
4. Give two investigations that may be performed in the acute phase of diverticulitis. **(2)**
5. Give one mainstay of the conservative management of diverticulitis. **(1)**
6. What are two possible complications of diverticulitis? **(2)**

**Q3** A 19-year-old man is seen by his GP for a swelling in his left groin. He noticed it shortly after he began going to the gym. On examination, a mass is palpable in the left groin, which has a cough impulse. The diagnosis of a left inguinal hernia is made.

1. What is the definition of a hernia? **(1)**
2. With relation to the pubic tubercle, how do you differentiate between inguinal and femoral hernias? **(1)**
3. With relation to the inferior epigastric vessels, how do you differentiate between indirect and direct inguinal hernias? **(1)**
4. Using embryology, explain how indirect inguinal hernias occur. **(2)**
5. Give two risk factors for inguinal hernias. **(2)**
6. What is the difference between an obstructed and a strangulated inguinal hernia? **(1)**
7. Give two complications following inguinal herniotomy surgery. **(2)**

**Q4** A 43-year-old woman presents to her GP with a 1-month history of fresh PR bleeding on defecation. Her perineum is examined, and she is found to have haemorrhoids.

1. What line divides internal and external haemorrhoids? **(1)**
2. Other than PR bleeding, give two symptoms of haemorrhoids. **(2)**
3. Name an investigation which may be performed. **(2)**
4. Give two conservative management options. **(2)**
5. Give two procedures which may be performed to manage haemorrhoids. **(2)**
6. Name one complication of haemorrhoids. **(1)**

**Q5** A 73-year-old lady is brought to A&E with acute severe central abdominal pain. However, on examination there are no abdominal signs. She is tachycardic and hypotensive. She has a history of AF. A diagnosis of acute mesenteric ischaemia is suspected.
1. Name the arterial supply to the foregut, midgut and hindgut. **(3)**
2. What acid-base disturbance is commonly associated with acute mesenteric ischaemia? **(1)**
3. Give two other abnormalities that may be found on blood tests. **(2)**
4. What is the gold standard for imaging in suspected acute mesenteric ischaemia? **(1)**
5. What are the aims of surgery for this condition? **(2)**
6. Give one essential component of the initial management prior to surgery. **(1)**

 **Q6** A 24-year-old male is brought into A&E after being stabbed in the left upper quadrant. He is haemodynamically unstable and a CT abdomen reveals a splenic injury. He undergoes an urgent splenectomy.
1. Name two other organs in the left upper quadrant that may have been damaged. **(2)**
2. What is the function of the red pulp of the spleen? **(1)**
3. What is the function of the white pulp of the spleen? **(1)**
4. Apart from trauma, give two indications for splenectomy. **(2)**
5. What type of organisms are people susceptible to following splenectomy? **(1)**
6. Due to people's susceptibility to these organisms, give two important aspects of long-term management following splenectomy. **(2)**

On a blood film following his splenectomy, the report mentions the presence of Howell–Jolly bodies.
7. What are Howell–Jolly bodies? **(1)**

**Q7** A 40-year-old man attends A&E with epigastric pain for the last 24 hours. The pain is getting worse and is radiating through to his back. He is finding it difficult to find any position that makes him feel comfortable and is sitting forward when you walk into the cubicle bay. He has recently split up from his partner and has found the break up difficult to deal with on top of recently being made unemployed. You suspect acute pancreatitis.

1. What is the most likely cause of this gentleman's pancreatitis? **(1)**
2. Name four other causes of pancreatitis. **(2)**
3. What blood test would confirm your suspicion? **(1)**
4. Name two potential early complications. **(2)**
5. Name two potential late complications. **(2)**
6. Describe the basis of the management. **(2)**

**Q8** A 58-year-old woman presents to A&E with a 1-day history of 'crampy tummy pains'. She hasn't opened her bowels since yesterday, and started vomiting this morning. She has undergone an appendicectomy and hysterectomy. She has hypertension and is taking ramipril. You suspect bowel obstruction.

1. What are the four main features of bowel obstruction? **(2)**
2. What features in a patient's history would make you think of small-bowel obstruction over large-bowel obstruction? **(2)**
3. Give four common causes of bowel obstruction. **(2)**
4. What clinical sign would distinguish between an ileus and a mechanical obstruction? **(1)**
5. What investigation would help you to distinguish between a small- and large-bowel obstruction? **(1)**
6. What immediate management would you start? **(2)**

**Q9**  A 40-year-old lady attends your GP clinic with epigastric pain, vomiting and fever which started this morning after waking. She has noticed that she has a crampy pain in the right upper quadrant after eating fatty meals for the last 2 months. On examination, she is Murphy's sign positive.

1. What is contained within bile? **(1 mark for each, max 2 marks)**
2. Name two types of gallstones based on composition. **(2)**
3. What are risk factors for developing gallstones? **(½ a mark for each, max 2 marks)**
4. What is Murphy's sign? **(2)**
5. What imaging would confirm the diagnosis of acute cholecystitis? **(1)**
6. What initial management would you start? **(1)**

**Q10** A 70-year-old man presents complaining of right upper quadrant pain, weight loss over the last 3 months and a reduction in his appetite. On examination, he has hepatomegaly and a hard discrete lump is felt along the border.

1. Name the four lobes of the liver. **(2)**
2. Which ligament divides the anterior of the liver into the two anterior lobes? **(1)**
3. Name three common origins of secondary tumour to the liver. **(3)**
4. Name three causes of hepatocellular carcinoma. **(3)**
5. What tumour marker is commonly raised in hepatocellular carcinoma? **(1)**

# Urology

Q1  Jim is a 72-year-old gentleman who has presented to A&E with a 24-hour history of increasing lower abdominal pain and anuria. On abdominal examination, he has a tender palpable bladder.

1.  List four causes of acute urinary retention. **(2)**
2.  Other than abdominal examination, name the other examination which should be performed and why. **(1)**
3.  He has a urinary catheter inserted in A&E. List two important things to undertake with regards to post-catheterisation care. **(2)**
4.  Blood is taken for urea and electrolyte analysis. List two other investigations which should be performed. **(1)**
5.  His potassium comes back as 6.8 mmol/L. List four treatments that may be started. **(2)**
6.  He initially drains 700 ml from his urinary catheter. Is this likely to be acute or chronic retention? **(1)**
7.  Although his pain is better after the catheter is inserted, Jim's catheter drains 500 ml of urine in the next 2 hours. What condition is Jim at risk of, and what precautions should be taken to treat this? **(2)**
8.  After correcting Jim's hyperkalaemia and fluid balance, his catheter is removed successfully. He is started on two medications during this admission. Name two medications he may have been started on, and how each of these medications exerts their effects. **(4 marks)**

**Q2** Joyce is a 67-year-old lady who has presented to your clinic with a 3-month history of intermittent painless macroscopic haematuria.

1. List four causes of macroscopic haematuria. **(2)**
2. List two investigations that would help establish a cause of Joyce's haematuria. **(2)**
3. List three factors that are associated with bladder tumours. **(2)**
4. She has a biopsy taken at cystoscopy, and there are malignant cells in her urine cytology. What is the most likely malignant cell in this patient – squamous cell, transitional cell or adenocarcinoma? **(1)**
5. Joyce's biopsy shows a T1 TCC of the bladder. What two treatments are indicated for this? **(2)**
6. List three places a bladder tumour may metastasise. **(3)**

**Q3** Sam is 66 years old and was referred to the urology clinic by his GP, as his PSA level was significantly raised.

1. List four non-malignant causes of a raised PSA. **(2)**

PSA has been considered to be used as a screening tool for prostate cancer.

2. Explain the following terms: sensitivity; positive predictive value **(2)**
3. What effect would a low PPV have on patients? **(1)**
4. List four criteria for a screening programme to be deemed suitable for a population. **(4)**
5. Sam is sent for a prostate biopsy and is given ciprofloxacin and metronidazole prior to the procedure. Why is antibiotic cover important for a prostate biopsy? **(1)**
6. Sam's biopsy results reveal a prostate adenocarcinoma. What score is used to evaluate prognosis? **(1)**
7. Sam undergoes active surveillance and hormonal treatment for his prostate cancer. Explain the term 'active surveillance'. **(1)**
8. List two treatments for more aggressive disease. **(1)**

**Q4** Tom is a 21-year-old medical student who has attended the A&E department with acute left-sided testicular pain that started an hour ago. He suffered a blow to the area in a rugby game. The A&E doctor is worried about testicular torsion.

1. List four other causes of testicular pain. **(2)**
2. What are the clinical features of testicular torsion? **(2)**
3. The surgical team review Tom and agree that testicular torsion is a possibility. What investigation is most likely and why? **(2)**
4. At operation, the scrotum is opened in layers to reach the testis. Name three layers. **(3)**
5. At operation, Tom undergoes a left orchidectomy and a right orchidopexy. Why does he undergo the second procedure at the same time? **(1)**
6. List two long-term sequelae of orchidectomy for testicular torsion. **(2)**

**Q5** Klaus, aged 55, comes to your clinic with a 4-month history of weight loss, haematuria and vague abdominal and back pain for the last 3 weeks. On examination, you find a left-sided mass.

1. What characteristics on examination would make you think this mass was renal in origin? **(2)**
2. Klaus undergoes further investigation and is found to have a malignant renal mass. What is the likely histology if Klaus was: 55 years old; 4 years old? **(2)**
3. On clinical investigation, Klaus has a painless testicular mass which feels like a 'bag of worms', especially when he stands up. What is the likely diagnosis and cause in this case? **(2)**
4. Routine blood tests for Klaus reveal the following results: Hb 17.8, WCC 6.8, Plts 234. Explain the abnormal Hb. **(1)**
5. List four risk factors for renal cell carcinoma. **(2)**
6. Klaus is considered for surgical intervention. What factors would affect his suitability for major surgery? **(2)**
7. Klaus undergoes a laparoscopic radial left nephrectomy. List two advantages of laparoscopic surgery over open surgery. **(2)**
8. List two disadvantages of laparoscopic surgery compared to open surgery. **(2)**

**Q6**  Rohit, aged 26, presented to the emergency department with a 24-hour history of colicky right-flank pain radiating to his groin.

1. Which bedside test would be useful in this situation? **(1)**
2. The admitting doctor thinks Rohit might have renal colic. What would be the radiological investigation of choice? **(1)**
3. Rohit's investigation shows a calculi obstructing the ureter. Why is pain referred to the groin? **(2)**
4. Why does ureteric obstruction cause pain? **(2)**
5. Where are three places the ureter is narrowed and more prone to obstruction with a stone? **(3)**
6. You are called to see Rohit because he has a fever of 39.2. What could be a source of Rohit's fever? **(1)**
7. Following ABC and initiating fluid resuscitation and antibiotics, what emergency intervention is indicated? **(1)**
8. Retrograde ureterogram and insertion of stent is used for patients with ureteric calculi. Why is this not indicated in this case? **(1)**
9. Name one lifestyle measure for the prevention of stones forming in the future. **(1)**

**Q7**  Jason, aged 5, is seen in clinic with his mother, with a painless scrotal swelling. On examination, it is separate from the testis.

1. What simple examination could help distinguish the cause? **(1)**
2. What radiological investigation could be used? **(1)**
3. Investigation is suggestive of hydrocoele. What is the anatomical basis of a hydrocoele? **(2)**
4. Hydrocoeles may be caused by other problems. List secondary causes of hydrocoele. **(2)**
5. Students are encouraged to make a 'triple diagnosis'. How would this apply to this case? **(3)**
6. Jason undergoes an excision and plication of hydrocoele. Why is the hydrocoele plicated? **(1)**
7. A hydrocoele found in infancy is indicative of what anatomical anomaly? **(1)**
8. What management is indicated if the patient is less than 1 year of age and why? **(2)**

**Q8**  Kenneth is due to undergo a TURP operation.

1.  Kenneth has the consent form explained to him. Name two general risks of an operation found on a consent form. **(2)**
2.  When counselling Kenneth about the operation, what two specific functions may he lose as a result of this operation? **(2)**
3.  Name two risks that are specific to TURP. **(2)**
4.  Kenneth is due to have his operation done under a spinal anaesthetic. What are two advantages of this method of anaesthetic compared with general anaesthetic? **(2)**
5.  Six hours after the operation, Kenneth has a seizure and difficulty breathing. He has no history of previous seizures and no co-morbid conditions. The doctor on call is worried about TURP syndrome. What is the mechanism by which TURP syndrome arises? **(2)**

**Q9** Maureen attends clinic with a long-standing history of urinary leaking when coughing, sneezing and laughing.

1.  Explain the following terms: stress incontinence; urge incontinence. **(2)**
2.  List two things that predispose to stress incontinence. **(2)**
3.  Maureen initially wishes to avoid surgical intervention for her incontinence. List four lifestyle changes or non-surgical methods that may help her incontinence. **(2)**
4.  A TVT procedure is performed. Maureen comes to clinic after her operation with improved stress incontinence, but still with symptoms of being 'caught short'. What psychological effects may this have on Maureen? **(1)**
5.  Oxybutinin is started. How does oxybutynin exert its effect? List three side effects. **(4)**

**Q10** Derek, aged 52, is referred to the urology department by his GP. This year, he has had four urinary tract infections (UTIs).

1. Name two causes of recurrent urinary tract infection in men. **(2)**
2. Name three common organisms found in UTI. **(3)**
3. You suspect Derek may have a urethral stricture. Name two causes of urethral stricture. **(2)**
4. Name one other clinical feature of urethral stricture. **(1)**
5. You decide to send Derek for a cystoscopy. List two other investigations for possible urethral stricture. **(2)**
6. Name two complications of urethral stricture. **(2)**
7. Cystoscopy reveals a stricture in the anterior urethra, and it also shows a large out-pouching of bladder mucosa. What is this and what has caused it? **(2)**
8. Name a treatment for urethral stricture. **(1)**

# Trauma and orthopaedics

**Q1** A 35-year-old man attends A&E with a painful right knee. It started hurting this morning and the pain has become worse. He is now unable to move his knee due to pain and it has become swollen and hot. He also complains of feeling hot. He has previously been fit and well. You suspect septic arthritis.

1. What is the most likely bacterial cause in an adult? **(1)**
2. What fluids will you send for culture? **(2)**
3. Name two other inflammatory markers that will be raised along with the white cell count. **(2)**
4. Outline your immediate management plan. **(2)**
5. Following your prompt orthopaedic referral, what may orthopaedics add to your management plan? **(1)**
6. What other organism should be considered if a metal prosthesis was in situ in the joint? **(1)**
7. Give two risk factors for developing septic arthritis. **(2)**

**Q2** A 60-year-old man tripped and fell up his front doorstep. He landed on his right elbow, and following this noticed some pain in his shoulder. He ignored it, and it settled down over the next few days, but he noticed it was more difficult than usual to move his arm. After a full shoulder examination, you feel he has a complete supraspinatus tendon tear.

1. Name the other rotator cuff muscles. **(3)**
2. Where does the supraspinatus attach to the humerus? **(1)**
3. What muscle takes over abduction of the arm after the supraspinatus initiates movement (the first 10–15 degrees of movement)? **(1)**
4. What two muscles are innervated by the accessory nerve? **(2)**
5. What two methods are used to image the supraspinatus and to assess whether any labral tears are present? **(2)**

3 You are working as an FY2 in accident and emergency. An ambulance phones through information on their transfer to the accident and emergency department and states: '24-year-old male, unrestrained driver in a 30-mph head-on collision, road traffic accident, blood pressure 105 over . . .' before the call is cut off. On arrival to the emergency department, the man is brought in unconscious and transferred onto the trolley on a spinal board with collar, blocks and tape immobilising his cervical spine. You perform a primary assessment of the patient by using a stepwise A, B, C, D, E approach. You start to assess his airway and you can hear a snoring-like sound coming from the airway.

1. What manoeuvre should you perform initially? **(1)**
2. What adjunct is available to help manage this patient's airway? **(1)**

You successfully manage to secure the airway. His respiratory rate is 20, oxygen saturations 96%, air entry is equal and vesicular breath sounds throughout the chest.

3. What can you do to improve this patient's 'breathing' and how would you do this? **(1)**

You move on to assess his circulation. He is tachycardic at 110, with a blood pressure of 90/60. There is no obvious site of bleeding on quick examination. His heart sounds are normal.

4. Give two initial steps you would take to manage his circulatory problems. **(2)**
5. What four urgent blood tests would you request at this point? **(2)**

You calculate his GCS as 6. His BM is 6.3.
6. Below what GCS is the airway at risk of not being maintained? **(1)**

His airway is temporarily being maintained with the simple adjunct you placed earlier, and you arrange with the nurse present to gather equipment to place a definitive airway. Whilst this is taking place, you examine his abdomen and feel an enlarged spleen.

7. You arrange for radiographs to be taken within the resuscitation room. Name two images you would request in a trauma series. **(2)**
8. What two forms of complex imaging would allow you to fully assess the extent of his injuries? **(2)**

**Q4** A 19-year-old male is brought into accident and emergency, having been stabbed outside a nightclub. He has a stab wound entering the right lower chest. He is breathing fast and is agitated. You perform a primary assessment of the patient by using a stepwise A, B, C, D, E approach. He is talking, but seems agitated. You are satisfied currently his airway is maintained. He is tachypnoeic with a respiratory rate of 28. His oxygen saturation is 88%. You ask the nurse to start 15 L of oxygen through a non-rebreathe mask. He has good air entry on the left side of his chest. You are unable to hear any air entry to the right side of his chest. You check his trachea; it is shifted to the left. You perform percussion of his chest.

1. The percussion was hyperresonant. What does this signify? **(1)**
2. How should this be managed acutely? Describe using precise anatomical landmarks. **(2)**
3. If percussion was dull on the right, what would this signify and how should this be managed acutely? **(2)**

You inspect the chest cavity, and there is a 3-cm laceration entering the chest wall around the 6th intercostal space.

4. Give two other structures that could be damaged and that are important to consider. **(2)**

The patient's saturations improve and his respiratory rate falls to 20. You move on to complete your survey. His heart sounds are normal, blood pressure 100/70 and heart rate 105. His GCS is 15, BM 5.9. His abdomen is soft and non-tender.

5. What initial imaging would you perform? **(1)**

The patient stabilises further following a bag of IV fluids and the acute management you performed.

6. What procedure needs to be performed for the next step in managing his condition? **(1)**

**Q5** A 17-year-old man was tackled whilst playing football. The other player landed on the lateral aspect of his left knee and 'pushed it inwards'. He has come straight to the accident and emergency department, and complains of pain and swelling of his left knee.

1. What test is performed to test the integrity of the anterior cruciate ligament? **(1)**
2. What test is performed to test the integrity of the posterior cruciate ligament? **(1)**
3. Describe how you test the collateral ligaments of the knee. **(2)**

Examination demonstrates a complete tear in the anterior cruciate ligament and the medial collateral ligament.

4. What is the third structure to be damaged with these two ligaments to make up the 'unhappy triad'? **(1)**
5. Why is this structure also commonly damaged? **(1)**
6. What test may be positive with a meniscal tear? **(1)**
7. What imaging can be used to assess the damage to the medial meniscus? **(1)**
8. Where can an autograft be taken from if the anterior cruciate ligment is to be reconstructed? **(1)**
9. If an arthroscopy to further assess the meniscus is undertaken, which cruciate ligament is seen attaching anteriorly to the tibial plateau? **(1)**

**Q6** An 81-year-old woman is brought into A&E after sustaining a fall. She is complaining of pain in her right hip. She is known to have osteoporosis. An AP and lateral X-rays of the right hip confirm a displaced intracapsular fracture of the neck of the femur.

1. What position would you expect see on inspection of the right leg? **(2)**
2. If X-rays are inconclusive, give an alternative imaging method which may be used to confirm a fractured neck of the femur. **(1)**
3. What system is used to classify intracapsular femoral neck fractures? **(1)**
4. Name two arterial supplies to the head of the femur. **(2)**
5. What complication may occur if the blood supply to the head of the femur is disrupted by an intracapsular fracture? **(1)**
6. What operative procedure will be performed if there is a displaced intracapsular fracture where there are concerns that the blood supply has been disrupted? **(1)**
7. What alternative procedure will be performed if there is an undisplaced intracapsular fracture and therefore the blood supply remains intact? **(1)**
8. Name one blood test which should be performed prior to surgery. **(1)**

**Q7** A 69-year-old lady attends A&E after sustaining a fall on her left hand. On inspection of the left arm, there is a 'dinner fork' deformity at the wrist. X-rays confirm a Colles' fracture.

1. What bone is fractured in a Colles' fracture? **(1)**
2. What part of the bone is fractured? **(1)**
3. What displacement and angulation of the distal fragment is present? **(1)**
4. What is the difference in a Smith's fracture? **(1)**

The orthopaedic registrar sees the patient in A&E and decides to reduce the fracture using a Bier's block.

5. Describe how a Bier's block is performed. **(2)**

After reduction is performed, a back-slab cast is applied.

6. What imaging should be performed after the back slab is applied and why? **(2)**
7. Give an operative procedure which may be performed if surgery is required. **(1)**
8. Approximately how long does a Colles' fracture take to heal? **(1)**

**Q8** A 27-year-old male is involved in a road traffic accident and sustains an open fractured left tibia and fibula. On admission to A&E, he is in severe pain and is tachycardic and hypotensive.

1. Define an open fracture. **(1)**
2. What system is used to classify open fractures? **(1)**
3. Give four components of managing an open fracture. **(4)**

The next day, following management of the open fracture, the patient is seen on the ward round. He is complaining of excruciating pain in the posterior aspect of his left lower leg which is exacerbated by dorsiflexion of the foot.

4. What complication is the patient experiencing? **(1)**
5. What is the surgical management of this condition? **(1)**
6. Apart from this complication, give two complications of an open fracture. **(2)**

**Q9** A 62-year-old woman with lower back pain and bilateral sciatica presents to her GP. On examination, there are bilateral lower motor signs in her lower limbs. Cauda equina syndrome is suspected.

1. What is the termination of the spinal cord known as? **(1)**
2. At what vertebral level does it occur in adults? **(1)**
3. At what vertebral level does it occur at in newborns? **(1)**
4. What are two possible causes of cauda equina syndrome? **(2)**
5. Give two lower motor neurone signs. **(2)**
6. What is the preferred imaging modality in suspected cauda equina syndrome? **(1)**
7. What is the definitive management of this condition? **(1)**
8. Give one potential complication if it is left untreated. **(1)**

**Q10** A 76-year-old woman with a 3-month history of pain in her left knee is seen by her GP. The GP suspects osteoarthritis.

1. What gender is more at risk of developing osteoarthritis? **(1)**
2. Give two features that may be found on examination of her left knee. **(2)**
3. What are the swellings at distal interphalangeal joints affected by osteoarthritis known as? **(1)**
4. What are the four changes that are typically seen on an X-ray of a joint affected by osteoarthritis? **(2)**
5. Give two pieces of lifestyle advice this patient may be given. **(2)**
6. Give two reasons to consider joint arthroplasty. **(2)**

# ENT

**Q1** A 93-year-old woman is admitted to A&E with significant epistaxis. She has hypercholesterolaemia, osteoarthritis and atrial fibrillation, she takes simvastatin, paracetamol, digoxin and warfarin.

1. What is the commonest cause of epistaxis? **(1)**
2. What is the name of the area on the anterior nasal septum where epistaxis commonly originates? **(1)**
3. Give two reasons why it is appropriate to do an FBC. **(2)**
4. Apart from an FBC, name two other blood tests which may be performed. **(2)**
5. Give two simple initial management steps. **(2)**
6. Give two methods by which the epistaxis may be stopped. **(2)**

**Q2** A 7-year-old boy presents to the urgent care centre with a 3-day history of sore throat and pain on swallowing. He is examined and found to have bilaterally inflamed tonsils and lymphadenopathy. A diagnosis of acute tonsillitis is made.

1. What is the medical term for pain on swallowing? **(1)**
2. Apart from a sore throat and pain on swallowing, what other symptoms may the patient be experiencing? **(2)**
3. What is the name of the lymph node commonly found to be enlarged in tonsillitis? **(1)**
4. Give two differentials for tonsillitis. **(2)**
5. If antibiotics are prescribed, why is penicillin V given as opposed to amoxicillin? **(1)**
6. Give two conservative management options which the parents will be advised about. **(2)**
7. One of the complications of acute tonsillitis is a peritonsillar abscess. What is the other name of this condition? **(1)**

**Q3** A 70-year-old man presents to A&E with difficulty swallowing. On further questioning, he tells you that he has difficulty swallowing solids but swallowing fluid is normal.

1. What is the medical term for difficulty swallowing? **(1)**
2. What is the significance of swallowing fluid being normal but swallowing solids being difficult? **(1)**

The gentleman undergoes an OGD and is found to have oesophageal carcinoma. Looking back in his medical notes, you find an OGD 5 years ago demonstrated Barrett's oesophagus.

3. What is Barrett's oesophagus? **(2)**
4. What type of oesophageal carcinoma does Barrett's oesophagus predispose somebody to? **(1)**
5. Apart from Barrett's oesophagus, give two other risk factors for oesophageal carcinoma. **(2)**
6. What staging system is used to stage oesophageal carcinoma? **(1)**
7. Give two possible treatment options for oesophageal carcinoma. **(2)**

**Q4** A 67-year-old lady is seen in the ENT outpatient clinic because of a hoarse voice. Vocal cord palsy secondary to recurrent laryngeal nerve palsy is suspected.

1. Which cranial nerve is the recurrent laryngeal nerve a branch of? **(1)**
2. Which side is recurrent laryngeal nerve palsy commoner on and why? **(2)**
3. What is the only laryngeal muscle not supplied by the recurrent laryngeal nerve, and what nerve is this muscle supplied by? **(2)**
4. Give two possible causes of recurrent laryngeal nerve palsy. **(2)**
5. Give two other symptoms of vocal cord palsy other than hoarseness. **(2)**
6. What procedure is used in the ENT outpatient setting to visualise the vocal cords? **(1)**

**Q5** A 54-year-old man attends your GP practice complaining that he woke up this morning with left-sided facial weakness. At breakfast this morning, he noticed he was dribbling his tea from the right side of his mouth and booked an emergency appointment straight after this. His wife is worried he has had a stroke.

1. List five other causes of unilateral facial weakness. **(2½)**
2. How can you discriminate an upper motor neurone lesion from a lower motor neurone lesion affecting the face? **(1)**
3. Name the five major branches of the facial nerve. **(2½)**
4. What treatments may you start? **(2)**
5. Give two long-term consequence of Bell's palsy. **(2)**

**Q6** A 70-year-old lady attends your GP clinic complaining of 'the room spinning' after turning her head right, which lasts around 30 seconds. This has been present for a few weeks now, and she has become fed up feeling like this. She denies tinnitus, and has not noticed her hearing change. A diagnosis of benign paroxysmal positional vertigo (BPPV) is made.

1. What is vertigo? **(1)**
2. Give four other causes of vertigo. **(2)**
3. Describe the pathogenesis of BPPV. **(2)**
4. What test is diagnostic of this condition? **(1)**
5. What manoeuvre can be used to treat this condition? **(1)**
6. How else could you manage this patient? **(3)**

**Q7** A 43-year-old woman attends your GP clinic with a 2-day history of pain in her left ear, fever and nausea. She has had a cough and coryzal symptoms for the last 3 days preceding this. She is otherwise fit and well, but does find juggling her job and caring for her three children difficult. You suspect otitis media.

1. What is otitis media? **(1)**
2. Name two common bacterial causes. **(2)**
3. How do children's Eustachian tubes differ in shape to adults', and what is the clinical consequence of this? **(2)**

You examine the tympanic membrane of the left ear.

4. Name the two portions of the eardrum. **(2)**
5. What might you find on otoscopy? **(3)**
6. What medication will you prescribe to manage this condition? **(2)**

**Q8** A 65-year-old man attends your GP clinic complaining that he feels his hearing has changed. His wife has noticed that sometimes he just ignores her when she speaks to him, and she has grown tired of having to shout to gain his attention. He has also started complaining of tinnitus. He has hypertension and hypercholesterolaemia, and is currently taking simvastatin and ramipril. He thinks he is allergic to shellfish. You perform hearing tests in your clinic. Rinne's test is positive in both ears. For Weber's test, the sound is heard loudest in the left ear.

1. What is the explanation for this finding? **(1)**
2. What tuning fork should be used to test hearing? **(1)**
3. Where is the tuning fork placed to elicit bone conduction in Rinne's test? **(1)**
4. What is a positive Rinne's test? **(1)**
5. What two possible consequences give a positive Rinne's test? **(2)**
6. How do you perform Weber's test? **(2)**

You suspect compression of the vestibulocochlear nerve, possibly by a vestibular schwannoma (acoustic neuroma).

7. Is a vestibular schwannoma benign or malignant? **(1)**
8. How do you confirm the diagnosis of vestibular schwannoma? **(1)**
9. What is the main differential diagnosis? **(1)**
10. What potential treatment option is available? **(1)**

**Q9** A 19-year-old attends A&E complaining of pain in her left cheek and dripping from her nose. She is normal, fit and well, and has just started university after a taking a gap year travelling America with a dance troupe. You suspect maxillary sinusitis.

1. What is a paranasal sinus? **(1)**
2. Name the paranasal sinuses. **(4)**
3. What epithelium lines the paranasal sinuses? **(1)**
4. Give two causes of maxillary sinusitis. **(2)**
5. How would you manage acute sinusitis? **(2)**

**Q10** A 60-year-old man attends your GP clinic complaining of a lump on the outer aspect of his cheek. He first noticed it a few months ago, but as it hasn't disappeared he wants your opinion on what it is. There is no pain associated with it, and he has not noticed any other swellings in his neck and feels otherwise well. Following examination, you feel that this swelling is within the parotid gland.

1. What cranial nerve would you examine? **(1)**
2. What are the other pairs of salivary glands? **(2)**
3. What percentage of tumours within the salivary glands are found in the parotid gland? **(1)**
4. What is the commonest tumour of the parotid gland? **(1)**
5. What features would lead you to expect a carcinoma? **(2)**
6. Where does the parotid duct enter the mouth? **(1)**
7. Excluding tumours, what other conditions can lead to unilateral swelling of the parotid gland? **(2)**

# Vascular

Q1  John, aged 65, has been sent a letter from his local hospital inviting him to attend the hospital for a USS as part of a local abdominal aortic aneurysm (AAA) screening.

1. What is the definition of an arterial aneurysm? **(1)**
2. What is the difference between a true aneurysm and a false aneurysm? **(1)**
3. Analysis of screening programs often quotes a 'number needed to screen'. What is the meaning of a 'number needed to screen'? **(1)**
4. Why may the number needed to screen be quite high in this case? **(1)**
5. John was found to have an AAA on USS screening of 6.0 cm diameter. What do you think the next step in John's management should be? **(1)**
6. Name two causes of an AAA. **(2)**
7. John goes to see a vascular surgeon about his AAA. His surgeon assesses his cardiovascular risk factors. List four cardiovascular risk factors. **(2)**
8. John decides to undergo an open repair of AAA. Name four possible complications of surgery that you must counsel John about. **(2)**
9. What factor may make John a candidate for endovascular aneurysm repair (EVAR) as opposed to open surgery? **(1)**
10. What are the possible disadvantages of using EVAR? **(2)**

**Q2** Barry, aged 72, is brought into A&E by ambulance with sudden-onset severe abdominal and back pain. Whilst in the ambulance, he collapsed, and on arrival has a BP of 80/50 and a pulse of 130. On examination, he has a tender expansile mass.

1. What important diagnosis must you consider at this point? **(1)**
2. Name two other diagnoses that could be considered in Barry's case. **(2)**
3. If the patient were stable, what diagnostic imaging could help in this case? **(1)**
4. Name two investigations important in this case. **(2)**
5. Barry is taken to theatre for an open repair of AAA using a Gore-Tex graft. He loses 4 L of blood intraoperatively. Name two blood products that Barry requires. **(2)**
6. Day 2 post-op, Barry is extubated on ITU. On examination of his feet, you notice mottled skin and darkened segments in his toes. What is this phenomenon's name and what is it due to? **(2)**
7. Going from innermost layer to outermost layer, name the four layers of an arterial vessel wall. **(2)**
8. Aneurysm formation occurs through a complex physiological process involving biomechanical forces, an immune response to cholesterol deposition, a shift towards proteolytic vessel wall remodelling and inflammation. Name a cell type that may be present in an aneurysmal wall. **(1)**

**Q3**  Fiona, aged 55, attends the emergency department of your district general hospital with sudden-onset severe lower left leg pain. Her left limb pulses are absent.

1.  What is the serious diagnosis to consider in this case? **(1)**
2.  Name four other symptoms that are associated with the condition named in 1. **(2)**
3.  What are the two commonest causes of the condition named in 1? **(1)**
4.  Fiona has recently been in hospital with newly diagnosed AF and has no previous history of claudication. What is the most likely cause of Fiona's current condition? **(1)**
5.  Your registrar feels that Fiona needs to be urgently transferred to a vascular surgery centre for definitive treatment. What two treatments can you institute in the interim? **(2)**
6.  Why must definitive treatment be performed urgently? **(1)**
7.  Name two possible definitive treatments for this condition. **(2)**
8.  Fiona goes to a vascular centre for surgical treatment. She has a continuous heparin infusion. Explain how heparin prevents blood clots. **(2)**
9.  Name two potential problems using a heparin infusion. **(2)**

**4** Ishant, aged 63, comes to your general practice as he is having trouble with walking. He says he can only walk 10 yards before having to stop. He has a background of GORD, hypertension, type 2 diabetes and hyperlipidaemia. He has a smoking history of 50 pack-years.

1. Ishant describes a burning pain in his left calf and thigh that develops when he walks 50 yards, causing him to stop and rest for 5 minutes until the pain goes away. What is the name given to this symptom? **(1)**

2. The symptom you named in the above question is a sign of which disease? What other diseases is he at risk of? **(3)**

3. What lifestyle management could you offer Ishant? **(1)**

4. What medical treatment could be beneficial for Ishant? **(2)**

5. Ishant tries conservative management and sees you again 3 months later. His symptoms have worsened. He now has pain at rest and has to hang his left leg out of bed at night to relieve his pain. What are these symptoms a sign of? **(1)**

6. Ishant has buttock pain and has recently developed impotence. Explain two possible locations of an arterial stenosis. **(2)**

7. What diagnostic investigation could Ishant undergo? **(1)**

8. Ishant undergoes an angioplasty + stenting to help a common iliac stenosis. Name one blood test that he must undergo before the procedure. **(1)**

9. A guide-wire is fed from arterial puncture in the common femoral artery into the aorta. List the arteries that the guide-wire must travel through. **(1)**

**Q5**  Valerie, aged 67, has come to A&E with a 30-minute history of left-sided weakness, speech slurring and blurred vision. These symptoms resolved whilst en route to the hospital.

1. What is the name for this collection of symptoms? **(1)**
2. This condition has a high incidence rate in acute hospitals. What does incidence rate mean? **(1)**
3. Why might incidence of this condition be decreasing? **(1)**
4. Valerie has blood tests and an ECG. What may an ECG reveal about the cause of Valerie's symptoms? **(1)**
5. Name two radiological investigations that are indicated in this case. **(2)**
6. Your consultant wants to assess Valerie's risk of future stroke and asks you assess her $ABCD^2$ score. What criteria make up the $ABCD^2$ score? **(2)**
7. Valerie tells you that about 6 months ago, she had a curtain fall over her left-eye vision which lasted for about 10 minutes. What is this phenomenon known as, and what causes it? **(2)**
8. Valerie has 75% stenosis of the right internal carotid artery. She is keen to undergo a carotid endarterectomy. Name two specific risks of the operation you should discuss. **(2)**
9. For the operation, an incision is made anterior to the sternomastoid and the carotid arteries are dissected and clamped. What structures are at risk of damage in this area? **(2)**
10. This procedure is increasingly done under regional anaesthetic. How may this be an advantage? **(1)**

**Q****6** Leslie, aged 59, comes to see you, as she has developed an ulcer on her left heel. She has a history of type 2 diabetes. She currently takes insulin, metformin and simvastatin.

1. What is the definition of an ulcer? **(1)**
2. List four possible vascular complications of long-term diabetes. **(2)**
3. List four causes of skin ulceration. **(2)**
4. Leslie's ulcer may be neuropathic, ischaemic or mixed. What factors would you use to distinguish neuropathy and ischaemia? **(3)**
5. What two things can help prevent Leslie developing further ulcers? **(2)**
6. Leslie is sent for an angiogram of her legs. Why must metformin be stopped for 48 hours prior to this? **(1)**
7. Later in the year, Leslie comes into the emergency department with a left-toe ulcer that has become increasingly painful and leaking offensive pus. What are the principles of management here? **(2)**
8. After treatment, Leslie's ulcer begins to heal by secondary intention. Explain the difference between primary and secondary intention. **(2)**

**Q7** Winifred, aged 70, is 5 days post–left total hip replacement. She complains of pain in her left leg.

1. What should be used for prevention of DVT in surgical patients at high risk of DVT? **(2)**
2. What are the clinical features of a unilateral DVT? **(2)**
3. Name four risk factors for DVT. **(2)**
4. A DVT may form due to impaired blood flow through a vessel. This is one part of Virchow's triad. What are the other two aspects of Virchow's triad? **(2)**
5. A blood test for D-dimers is sent. Why should this test be used with caution in DVT? **(1)**
6. What investigation is warranted if pelvic or lower-limb DVT is suspected? **(1)**
7. Winifred's ultrasound shows a likely DVT in the left femoral vein. What treatments are indicated in the short term and the long term? **(2)**
8. What are two possible complications of complete DVT? **(2)**
9. Winifred has ongoing problems with recurrent complications of DVT, despite being on oral anticoagulation therapy. What further mechanical treatment may be possible? **(1)**

**8** John aged, 64, is due to have a right below-knee amputation for gangrene of his first three toes secondary to severe arterial disease of his right leg.

1. List two other indications for an amputation. **(2)**
2. When planning for this surgery, what is important to consider with regards to the level of amputation? **(2)**
3. Name two examples of each of the following that are transected in a below-knee amputation: bones, arteries and muscles. **(3)**
4. Immediately before the operation, whilst checking John's consent, what else is it important to ensure with regard to operative site? **(1)**
5. Two days after the operation, John's patient-controlled analgesia (PCA) is ceased. He complains of burning pain where his limb used to be. What is the name of this phenomenon and what is its basis? **(2)**
6. What sort of medical treatments are available for neuropathic pain? **(1)**
7. List two other complications specific to an amputation. **(2)**
8. After the amputation, the stump undergoes a dynamic process of wound healing. Broadly, what are the main stages of the model of wound healing? **(2)**

 **9** Deborah, aged 42, visits her GP with a complaint of unsightly bumps on her legs. It appears she has varicose veins.

1. How do varicose veins arise? **(2)**
2. List two risk factors for varicose veins. **(1)**
3. Most varicose veins are idiopathic. Name two conditions that may cause varicose veins. **(2)**
4. On examination, what skin changes would you look for? **(2)**
5. Another aspect of examination is testing the saphenovenous junction. How is this located? **(1)**
6. What non-medical interventions could you advise Deborah of? **(2)**
7. What complications may arise in long-term varicose veins? **(2)**
8. Deborah undergoes saphenofemoral ligation and long saphenous stripping with multiple avulsions. What nerve could get damaged and what symptoms would this produce below the knee? **(2)**

Q10 Stephen, aged 22, has been brought into A&E following a stab wound to the right groin in an alleged assault. He is bleeding profusely from a wound in his groin.

1. What are the first three things to assess in this emergency situation? **(3)**
2. What can be done immediately for a life-threatening wound? **(1)**
3. On secondary survey, the surgical team describe the wound as being in the 'femoral triangle'. What are the boundaries of the femoral triangle? **(3)**
4. What structures are at risk from an injury to this region? **(2)**
5. What other signs on examination suggest a vascular injury? **(2)**
6. Stephen undergoes urgent surgical repair of a femoral artery laceration. What investigation can check the repair was successful? **(1)**
7. What complications can arise from a vascular injury? **(1)**
8. Twelve hours post-op, Stephen complains of excruciating pain in his right leg, out of proportion to the injury he sustained. What surgical emergency must you consider and what treatment is indicated? **(2)**

# Clinical specialties

# Dermatology

**Q1** A mother brings her 7-year-old boy to you in the GP surgery, telling you he is constantly scratching at the back of his knee. You suspect eczema.

1. What is the usual distribution of atopic eczema? **(1)**
2. Name two other clinical conditions that can be present in people who suffer eczema as part of atopy. **(2)**
3. Describe the classical findings of eczema on examination. **(3)**

On examination, as well as the findings you have described above, you find some yellow exudate at the pruritic sites. You think it may be infected.

4. What is the most likely organism group causing the infection? **(1)**
5. Other than topical steroids and emollients, name two other therapies that can be used to treat eczema. **(2)**
6. What serum immunoglobulin is usually elevated in patients who suffer from severe eczema? **(1)**

**Q2** A 22-year-old man presents with a 'rash' on his elbow.

1. State four questions you would ask in the history. **(2)**

After taking a history and examining the patient, you are sure that it is plaque psoriasis.

2. What is the classical appearance of plaque psoriasis? **(2)**
3. Name two other forms of psoriasis. **(2)**
4. Other than the lesion site he shows you, where else should you examine? Name two sites. **(1)**
5. State four treatments that can be used for plaque psoriasis. **(2)**
6. What is the Koebner phenomenon? **(1)**

**Q3** A 20-year-old Ashkenazi Jewish gentleman comes to see you looking very unwell. He is complaining of blisters erupting all over his body, particularly in the mouth, that are easily burst, and most appear loose on examination.

1. What is the likely diagnosis? **(2)**
2. What is the medical term for large blister? **(1)**
3. What tests would you order? **(2)**
4. What in general terms are the two possible causes of the disorder you have identified? **(2)**
5. What is Nikolsky's sign? **(2)**
6. In general terms, what is the treatment for this condition? **(1)**

**Q4** A 27-year-old girl comes to you in the GP practice complaining of an 'enlarging mole' on her neck.

1. State four questions you would want to ask about this 'mole'? **(2)**
2. Other than sun exposure, give two risk factors for developing malignant melanoma. **(2)**
3. Name two types of malignant melanoma. **(2)**
4. What is the most significant feature of a malignant melanoma in predicting prognosis? **(1)**
5. Name two other sites at which malignant melanoma can occur. **(2)**
6. What is the mainstay of treatment for these lesions? **(1)**

**Q5** A 37-year-old semi-professional golf player comes to see you in the GP surgery complaining of a hard skin lesion on his face. After taking a history and examining the patient, you believe this to be most likely a basal cell carcinoma (BCC).

1. Give three possible differential diagnoses of a BCC. **(3)**
2. What is the characteristic appearance of a BCC? Give three features. **(3)**
3. In this patient's case, what do you believe to be the most likely aetiological factor? **(1)**
4. What is the best surgical technique used to give the best cure rate for BCC? **(1)**
5. What will you advise this man to prevent recurrence of BCC? **(2)**

**Q6** A 17-year-old girl comes to the general dermatology clinic after referral from her GP for 'uncontrollable' acne. The patient is very upset and embarrassed about her condition, she is sometimes not going to college and spends most nights in rather than socialising with her friends.

1. Except for the face, where else does acne occur commonly? Name two sites. **(1)**
2. What is the pathophysiology of acne? **(2)**
3. What is the bacteria species that is commonly involved in the pathogenesis? **(1)**
4. Before talking about treatment, how will you educate and advise her about acne? Name one point. **(1)**
5. Except for isotretinoin, name one topical treatment option and one systemic treatment option for this patient. **(2)**
6. Name two common side effects of isotretinoin. **(2)**
7. What will you strongly advise her about when prescribing isotretinoin? **(1)**

**Q7** A 67-year-old gentleman comes into the GP surgery complaining of a persistent crusty lesion on the back of his right hand that is getting in the way of his gardening, which he likes to do all the time. He is usually fit and well, but has been taking life slowly since his kidney transplant 7 years ago. After examination, it is likely a squamous cell carcinoma (SCC).

1. Give three differential diagnoses of an SCC. **(3)**
2. What is the common name for carcinoma in situ of SCC called? **(1)**
3. What are the two big risk factors for SCC in this patient's case? **(2)**
4. What two anatomical sites on the head and neck give a worse prognosis? **(2)**
5. Where else would you examine other than the lesion site? Name one site. **(1)**
6. What would be the best treatment for this gentleman? **(1)**

**Q8** An 80-year-old male who is usually fit and well comes to see you in the GP surgery complaining of a 24-hour history of feeling generally unwell, with moderate to severe pain and burning sensation with an associated rash in the region from the left side of his back to his umbilicus, stopping in the midline.

1. What is the characteristic appearance of shingles? Name two salient points. **(2)**
2. What dermatome has been affected in this patient? **(1)**
3. What virus causes shingles? **(1)**
4. Name two groups of patients who are more susceptible to contracting shingles. **(2)**
5. Name two categories of drugs you would prescribe this gentleman. **(2)**
6. What is the commonest chronic complication of shingles? **(1)**
7. What is Ramsay Hunt syndrome? **(1)**

**Q9** You are the junior doctor on the stroke ward and you have been called to see Doreen, a 78-year-old who has had a dense left hemiparesis for the past 4 weeks. The nurse wants you to have a look at a wound on Doreen's sacral area.

1. What are the four grades of pressure sores? Describe the basic characteristic of each grade. **(4)**
2. Name four risk factors for developing a pressure sore. **(2)**

You inspect the wound and find it to be a grade-three pressure sore.

3. Name four points you could address in your management of Doreen's pressure sore. **(4)**

**Q10** A 57-year-old lady comes into your GP practice complaining of a skin lesion around her anogenital region. It appears as a white atrophic area and is itchy. You are confident this is a case of lichen sclerosus.

1. Give three differential diagnoses other than lichen sclerosus. **(3)**
2. Name two other symptoms or signs she may complain of. **(2)**
3. Name one investigation you would order. **(1)**
4. How would you treat this patient? Name two points. **(2)**
5. Name two complications of lichen sclerosus. **(2)**

# Ophthalmology

**Q1** A mother brings her 9-year-old son into the GP practice to see you. She tells you that her son has developed bilateral red itchy eyes, with some sticky exudate coming from both of them. You suspect conjunctivitis.

1. In very general terms, what can cause conjunctivitis? **(2)**
2. Give three other important causes of a red eye. **(3)**
3. What is the name of the eye-drop medication you will prescribe this patient? **(1)**
4. What general advice will you give to the patient and his mother? **(1)**
5. If these symptoms occurred in a neonate, what important causal organism should you consider? **(1)**

You have a medical student in with you, and you decide to let her do a full ophthalmological exam on the patient. The patient finds it very painful and uncomfortable to have the light shined in their eye. The medical student discloses to you that there was absence of the red-light reflex in the patient's left eye.

6. What is the term given for what the patient experienced whilst being examined? **(1)**
7. With regards to absence of red reflex, what important diagnosis must you consider? **(1)**

**Q2** A 64-year-old gentleman with long-term type 2 diabetes comes to see you in the routine ophthalmology clinic for annual review. One of the signs you see on the retina is a 'cotton wool spot' and small new vessels around the optic disc area.

1. What stage of diabetic retinopathy is described with the above findings? **(1)**
2. Name three other possible findings on the retina of this gentleman. **(3)**
3. What is a cotton wool spot? **(1)**
4. What treatment is this gentleman in need of? **(1)**
5. The patient also complains of gradual deterioration of the centre of his vision. What do you expect is happening? **(1)**
6. Name two other eye conditions that diabetic patients are at increased risk of. **(2)**
7. What is the best way of preventing diabetic retinopathy occurring? **(1)**

**Q3** A 74-year-old man who comes into your GP practice is found to have a blood pressure of 178/109 mmHg. You decide to investigate further and perform fundoscopy.

1. How is the severity of hypertensive retinopathy classified? **(1)**
2. Name four findings on the retina that are characteristic of severe hypertensive retinopathy. **(4)**
3. You see changes consistent with grade 2 hypertensive retinopathy. What are these changes? **(2)**
4. Given this patient's age, what is the first-line type of antihypertensive medication that should be given? **(1)**

The next patient has a similar presentation, with a blood pressure of 238/122 mmHg, but is complaining of blurred vision and palpitations. On fundoscopy, you notice an absence of venous pulsation, blurring of the disc margins and also a slight elevation of the disc bilaterally.

5. What ophthalmological sign are the above findings a description of? **(1)**
6. What endocrinological disease do you think might be causing this patient's severe hypertension? **(1)**

**Q4** Doris, a 77-year-old lady, comes to you in the GP surgery stating she is losing her vision.

1. State six questions you would want to ask Doris in order to try and find a cause of this loss in vision. **(3)**

After questioning, you suspect cataract.

2. Name two differential diagnoses other than cataract for loss of vision. **(1)**
3. Name two risk factors for the development of cataracts. **(2)**
4. Name one positive finding you will look for on examination. **(1)**
5. What is the surgical procedure used for the treatment of cataracts? **(1)**
6. Name the commonest early complication and the commonest late complication of the surgical procedure you have named above. **(2)**

**Q5** Richard, a 52-year-old taxi driver, comes to see you in the eye casualty with a presenting symptom of a 'sausage-shaped' visual loss in his right eye. You measure the intraocular pressure to be 32 mmHg. You suspect glaucoma.

1. What is used to measure intraocular pressure, and what is the upper limit of normal in mmHg? **(2)**
2. What is gonioscopy, and why is it important in this clinical case? **(2)**

You now suspect open-angle glaucoma.

3. What is the most important structure to now examine, and what will you look for? **(1)**
4. Name two common risk factors for open-angle glaucoma? **(2)**
5. Name four medical treatments that can be used to treat this patient? **(2)**
6. If his vision deteriorates, what organisation will you advise Richard to get in contact with? **(1)**

**Q6** A usually fully independent elderly lady comes to see you, guided by her daughter, in the ophthalmology outpatients' department. She complains of an acute visual disturbance. She describes 'lamp posts and door frames looking wiggly'. You suspect age-related macular degeneration (ARMD).

1. What type of ARMD do you suspect most? **(1)**
2. What investigations or examinations would you need to perform? Name two. **(2)**
3. When investigating the macular area of the retina, what is characteristically found in the type of ARMD you have mentioned above? Name two points. **(2)**
4. What management options are available for the type of ARMD you described above? **(3)**
5. What counselling or advice will you offer any patient with either form of ARMD? Name two points. **(2)**

**Q7** A 54-year-old gentleman comes to the emergency eye department complaining of an acutely painful right eye associated with a headache, vomiting and blurring of vision. He also states he had a similar episode in the past which resolved when he went to bed and fell asleep. You suspect acute angle-closure glaucoma (AACG).

1. State one risk factor for this condition. **(1)**
2. State four positive features you would expect to find on examination of this patient. **(4)**
3. How do you account for the blurred vision? **(1)**
4. How do you account for the previous episode resolving when going to bed? **(1)**
5. Name two agents you might use in your immediate management. **(2)**
6. What is the definitive treatment for this condition? **(1)**

**8** An 18-year-old comes into the eye casualty with two police guards after admitting to being in a fight. He complains of painless loss of vision in his right eye. Retinal detachment is at the top of your differential list.

1. State three other causes for sudden painless loss of vision. **(3)**

Retinal detachment is diagnosed, and after visual field testing, he has a loss of the upper half of his visual field in his right eye.

2. State the area of the retina that must be detached. **(1)**
3. Other than visual field loss, name two other symptoms he may be complaining of. **(2)**
4. Between people who have myopia and people who have hypermetropia, who are at the greater risk of retinal detachment? Explain your answer. **(2)**
5. Name two options for treatment for retinal detachment. **(2)**

**9** Pauline, an 80-year-old lady comes to see you in the eye casualty department. She is known to have polymyalgia rheumatica, but over the past few days she has been struggling with a right-sided headache in the temporal region which was associated with jaw claudication. Today, she lost her vision in her right eye 45 minutes ago. After examination, you are highly suspicious of a central retinal artery occlusion.

1. Name four steps in the general examination of a patient's eyes. **(2)**
2. Other than examining Pauline's eyes, name two other parts of your general examination that you would want to perform when high suspicion of central retinal artery occlusion is present. **(2)**
3. In general terms, what is the commonest cause of central retinal artery occlusion? **(1)**
4. What do you think the underlying pathological cause of her visual loss is? **(1)**
5. What will you find on testing the pupillary responses? **(1)**
6. What is the classical finding on fundoscopy of central retinal artery occlusion? **(1)**
7. What would be the immediate management of this patient? **(1)**
8. Is Pauline's sight salvageable in the time frame you have seen her? Yes/No **(1)**

Q10 A 77-year-old lady comes into the eye casualty after urgent referral from the GP with classical dermatological findings of ophthalmic shingles. The vesicular rash spreads to the tip of the patient's nose.

1. What virus causes shingles? **(1)**
2. What symptoms may the patient have had prior to the eruption of the shingles rash? Name two. **(1)**
3. Describe the usual distribution of any shingles infection. **(1)**
4. What nerve has been affected by the shingles to cause lesions extending down to the tip of the patient's nose? What is the significance of this? And what is this sign called? **(3)**
5. What chemical agent is used to visualise any ulceration of the cornea? **(1)**
6. What is the classical shape of the ulcers that form on the cornea in ophthalmic shingles? **(1)**
7. What is vital to test for as part of your eye examination in ophthalmic shingles and why? **(2)**

# Obstetrics

Q1 A 28-year-old parity 3 lady who is at 29 weeks' gestation comes to the emergency clinic complaining of finding a pool of blood on her bed sheets when she woke up this morning. She is slightly tachycardic at 103 bpm, but other observations are stable. On palpation, the foetal head is not engaged and high-lying. You suspect placenta praevia.

1. Name two situations where placenta praevia is more commonly found. **(2)**
2. What is the definition of antepartum haemorrhage? **(1)**
3. Name two other causes of antepartum haemorrhage. **(2)**
4. Why is vaginal examination never performed in a large antepartum haemorrhage? **(1)**
5. Name three investigations you would perform/request? **(3)**

She is rhesus negative.

6. What treatment would you administer? **(2)**

**Q2** A 27-year-old nulliparous lady who is at 31 weeks' gestation is admitted after some vaginal blood loss. Your consultant diagnoses on clinical grounds that she has a placental abruption.

1. Except vaginal blood loss, what is likely to be the most prominent symptom that the patient will be complaining of? **(1)**
2. What is placental abruption? **(1)**
3. What do you expect the lie and presentation to be in placental abruption? **(1)**
4. Name two major risk factors for placental abruption. **(1)**
5. She is tachycardic and hypotensive, but only a small amount of blood loss was seen from the vagina. How can these signs be explained? **(2)**
6. The mother is now stable after fluid resuscitation, steroids and anti-D have been administered, but your consultant believes the foetus to be in distress. What is the next major management step? **(1)**
7. What would you expect to see on clotting studies after a major abruption? Explain your answer. **(2)**
8. What is vasa praevia? **(1)**

**Q3** A 23-year-old Afro-Caribbean lady comes to see you complaining of missing her last three menstrual periods. The first day of her last menstrual period was 14 February. On examination of the abdomen, an enlarged uterus is palpated. You do a pregnancy test, and it is positive.

1. What component in urine is being measured when testing for pregnancy? **(1)**
2. What is the earliest (in weeks) a pregnant uterus can be palpated if there is a single foetus present? **(1)**
3. If she has a normal 28-day cycle, using Naegele's rule, when is her estimated due date? **(1)**
4. Name four blood tests that would be routinely offered to this woman. **(2)**

She states that she is unsure of the father as she has had multiple sexual partners over the last 6 months.

5. What screening will you now offer her and why? **(2)**
6. At the 11- to 14-week scan, there is increased nuchal translucency thickness. Except Down's syndrome, what can this be suggestive of? **(1)**
7. She is very anxious that her baby will have Down's syndrome, so you offer her the 'triple test'. Name two components of blood that are measured in the triple test and state whether they are normally increased or decreased if the child is suggestive of having trisomy 21? **(2)**

**Q4** A 28-year-old gravida 2 parity 1 attends your clinic after the midwife had repeated positive urine dipstick tests for glucose. An oral glucose tolerance test was performed prior to clinic, and it confirmed gestational diabetes. She had not been known to have diabetes prior to becoming pregnant.

1. Name three risk factors for developing gestational diabetes? **(3)**
2. Explain the mechanism behind the development of a macrosomic baby in diabetic pregnant women? **(2)**
3. Name risks to the foetus in women who suffer diabetes (gestational or established) during pregnancy? **(2)**
4. What is the commonest complication in the neonate post-delivery? **(1)**

She is worried that she may suffer diabetes in the future.

5. What will you tell this lady? **(2)**

**Q5** You are called to see a 21-year-old girl who is post-partum after a normal vaginal delivery. The midwife tells you she is accusing the staff of trying to kill her newborn child and her boyfriend is plotting with her mother to steal her child.

1. What is the diagnosis? **(1)**
2. What is the usual time frame from delivery to onset of this problem? **(1)**

Her boyfriend is worried about her future mental health and whether it will happen again in future pregnancies.

3. What will you tell him? **(2)**
4. Over what post-partum period does post-partum depression usually present? **(1)**
5. Approximately what percentage of pregnant women does post-partum depression affect? **(1)**
6. Name two maternal risk factors for developing post-partum depression. **(2)**
7. What medical diagnosis should be considered in women presenting with depressive symptoms post-partum? **(1)**
8. Regarding 'baby blues', apart from psychosocial factors, what is the probable cause? **(1)**

**Q6** A 21-year-old nulliparous lady comes to see you in the maternal assessment clinic after her midwife noted her blood pressure to be 149/106 and there was protein++ in her urine. She is otherwise well and has no symptoms. You suspect pre-eclampsia.

1. What is pre-eclampsia? **(1)**
2. Name six risk factors for the development of pre-eclampsia. **(3)**
3. Name four signs and symptoms of severe pre-eclampsia. **(2)**
4. Name two common antihypertensive drugs safely used in pregnancy for this lady. **(1)**

The patient's blood pressure rises to 211/129 on the next measurement, and she begins to have a seizure. The consultant identifies that the patient is having an eclamptic seizure.

5. What drug should be given now? Name the common method of monitoring its toxicity. **(2)**
6. What is HELLP syndrome? **(1)**

**Q7** An 18-year-old girl presents to the maternity assessment clinic stating that her 'waters have broken'. She is 27 weeks' pregnant. The midwife places her on the cardiotocograph and explains there is no uterine activity demonstrated on the print out.

1. What is the term used to describe the situation above? **(1)**
2. Name two specific drugs you would want to administer this patient. **(2)**
3. Name one maternal and foetal sign of chorioamnionitis. **(2)**

An identical case with similar cardiotocographic findings comes into the assessment centre; however, she is 38 weeks' pregnant and has no further contractions over the next 24 hours.

4. What would be the next reasonable course of action? **(1)**
5. Name the five components of the Bishop score. **(5)**
6. What is the first-line pharmacological method for aiding cervical ripening? **(1)**

**Q8** A 29-year-old gravida 7 para 2 who is 34 weeks' pregnant presents with acute-onset shortness of breath. On further questioning, she has a history of four previous miscarriages and pre-eclampsia in her last two successful pregnancies and is taking aspirin daily but can't remember why. You suspect a pulmonary embolism.

1. Name four other signs you should look for on history or examination of this woman. **(2)**

After a full examination, you are highly suspicious of a pulmonary embolism. The patient remains stable with a partial pressure of oxygen of 8.7 kPa on arterial blood gas sampling which increases to 10.9 kPa after administration of 8 L of oxygen via face mask.

2. What is your next step in the management of this patient? **(1)**
3. What test will you order to diagnose the suspected pulmonary embolism? **(1)**
4. Why do you suspect this patient is taking daily aspirin during her pregnancy? **(1)**
5. Name three pre-existing risk factors for venous thromboembolism in any patient? **(3)**
6. Why is deep vein thrombosis commoner in the left leg than the right leg in pregnant women? **(2)**

**9** A 27-year-old lady presents to you in the maternity assessment centre complaining of itching. She is 31 weeks' pregnant and is complaining of severe itching, particularly on the palms of her hands and soles of her feet. Her first two pregnancies ended in early miscarriage, the third was a successful pregnancy delivering by Caesarean section secondary to an estimated foetal weight of 4.8 kg and the most recent ended in stillbirth at 38 weeks' gestation. You suspect possible obstetric cholestasis.

1. What is her gravidy and parity? (answers as $G_xP_y$) **(1)**
2. Name the two most useful blood tests to do in this lady. **(2)**
3. What in her past obstetric history makes you suspicious she may have had obstetric cholestasis in the past? **(1)**
4. What are the risks of obstetric cholestasis? **(2)**
5. Name two pharmacological methods of treating obstetric cholestasis. **(2)**
6. What is the usual definitive management of obstetric cholestasis? **(1)**

Some weeks later, she gives birth to a healthy baby boy. She then returns to you and asks if she is likely to suffer with this again in future pregnancies?

7. What will you say to her? **(1)**

**Q10** You are the registrar on the labour ward. An alarm bell has been triggered in a room. On arrival, you can see a midwife and woman in labour. There is a baby's head at the vaginal introitus and it isn't moving. The midwife says, 'The baby is turtle-necking'. You believe that shoulder dystocia is occurring.

1. Name two pre-labour and two intra-partum risk factors for shoulder dystocia. **(2)**
2. What would be your first- and second-line manoeuvres to help the delivery of this child? **(2)**

The baby is eventually born after a simple manoeuvre. The baby is whisked away, and the midwife does a simple Apgar score on the child.

3. Name the five components of the Apgar score. **(5)**

You are called to another emergency in another room, You enter the room and see the midwife with her hand inside a labouring woman's vagina. She says, 'Cord prolapse, about 7 centimetres dilated!'

4. Name four risk factors for cord prolapse. **(2)**
5. What do you think the midwife is actively doing with her hand inside the patient's vagina? **(1)**
6. What is the definitive management step in this lady? **(1)**

**Q11** A patient comes to see you in the antenatal clinic after having a blood test due to feeling tired during pregnancy. She is 32 weeks' pregnant. The result is below:

Hb 10.8 g/dL (normal range 11.5–13.5)

MCV 90 fL (normal range 80–95)

1. Is this haemoglobin level normal for this patient? Explain your answer. **(2)**

You decide to examine her and you hear an ejection systolic murmur.

2. Should you be worried about finding this? Explain your answer. **(2)**

3. How do women increase their oxygen intake during pregnancy? **(1)**

You are then called to the maternity assessment centre to review a cardiotocograph on a lady who is complaining of tightenings.

4. What are the four parameters of a cardiotocograph trace that represent a reasurring trace? **(2)**

The trace showed some variable decelerations, and this prompted you to do a foetal blood sampling.

5. Name two contraindications to doing foetal blood sampling. **(2)**

6. Above what value is considered normal for foetal pH? **(1)**

# Gynaecology

Q1  Amanda, aged 22, presents to the emergency department with severe right lower quadrant pain.

1. Name two common causes of severe right lower abdominal pain other than ectopic pregnancy. **(2)**
2. Name two symptoms or signs that may make ectopic pregnancy more likely. **(2)**
3. What bedside investigation may help the diagnosis? **(1)**
4. Amanda is haemodynamically stable. What investigation is indicated? **(1)**
5. Name two factors predisposing to ectopic pregnancy. **(2)**
6. Name two sites where a fertilised ovum may implant. **(2)**
7. Investigations reveal an 8-week gestational sac in the right Fallopian tube. How could this patient be managed surgically? **(1)**
8. How could this case be managed medically, provided ectopic is small with minimal symptoms? **(1)**
9. Amanda's blood results come back: Hb 12.3; WCC 9.4; platelets 189; blood group A, rhesus negative. What further treatment is necessary after assessing the above bloods? **(1)**

**Q2** A 17-year-old girl in her 10th week of her first pregnancy comes to see you in the gynaecology emergencies clinic presenting with persistent vomiting for 10 days. She has been unable to keep any solids or fluids down for the past 2 days.

1. What is the likely diagnosis? **(1)**
2. Name three risk factors for developing this. **(3)**
3. What is the most important bedside investigation to perform, and what will you be looking for? **(1)**
4. Name two blood tests you would perform. **(1)**

Your registrar tells you to start her on some vitamin supplements.

5. Which vitamin will you prescribe, and what is the rationale behind this? **(2)**
6. Name two other treatments you may want to give a patient with this condition. **(1)**

An ultrasound scan was performed on this patient by your consultant because her uterus was found to be large for dates, and the image showed a 'snowstorm' appearance.

7. What is the likely diagnosis from the ultrasound scan? **(1)**

 **Q3** Shelley, aged 24, is 8 weeks into her third pregnancy. She comes to the emergency department with vaginal bleeding and lower abdominal pain.

1. Define the following terms: missed miscarriage, incomplete miscarriage, inevitable miscarriage. **(3)**
2. What two blood investigations should you perform? **(2)**
3. List three management options that are available to Shelley if incomplete miscarriage is confirmed. **(3)**
4. Shelley's bleeding continues, and a USS shows retained products of conception. She undergoes evacuation of retained products. Name an investigation that could occur with foetal products? **(1)**
5. What are two possible complications of surgical evacuation of the uterus? **(2)**
6. Name three causes of recurrent spontaneous miscarriage. **(3)**

**Q4** Susan, a 41-year-old smoker, comes to see you complaining of very heavy painful periods, with 7 days of bleeding including passing of clots.

1. Name three causes of menorrhagia. **(3)**
2. Susan is sent for full blood count, TFTs and clotting studies. Name two further investigations for menorrhagia. **(2)**
3. Susan is currently taking the combined oral contraceptive pill (COCP), but has been advised to stop as she is a smoker. List two other contraindications to taking the COCP. **(2)**
4. You think Susan has dysfunctional uterine bleeding. Name a medication that could reduce Susan's heavy bleeding. **(1)**
5. Susan feels she has completed her family and would like a hysterectomy. What two other procedures could you offer her before hysterectomy? **(2)**
6. Susan still opts for a hysterectomy. List two possible complications of a hysterectomy. **(2)**
7. What serious diagnosis is possible in post-menopausal bleeding? **(1)**

 **Q5** Deborah, aged 25, has been sent a letter inviting her to take part in the national cervical screening programme.

1. What micro-organism is implicated in cervical cancer? **(1)**
2. Name two risk factors for cervical cancer. **(2)**
3. Deborah has a cervical smear. The cytology shows moderate dyskaryosis. What investigation should she be referred for? **(1)**
4. On examination, you see ectropion. Explain the term ectropion. **(1)**
5. Name a cause of ectropion. **(1)**
6. Biopsy reveals a CIN III. Explain what CIN III is. **(2)**
7. What procedure can be used to completely remove CIN III? **(1)**
8. Deborah comes to her follow-up 6 months later, complaining of post-coital bleeding, and has a further biopsy. Name the two histological types of cervical cancer. **(2)**
9. Deborah's second biopsy shows invasive carcinoma. What investigation could be used to assess local and distant spread? **(1)**

**Q6** Kerry, aged 44, presents to the emergency department with severe left lower quadrant pain.

1. List two gynaecological causes of acute left lower abdominal pain. **(2)**
2. Name two investigations for assessing your answers to 1. **(2)**
3. What are the clinical features of ovarian torsion, and how does it arise? **(2)**
4. A solid cystic mass is found on the left ovary, with calcified structures that look similar to teeth. What is the diagnosis? **(1)**
5. How does the answer you gave in the above question arise? **(1)**
6. Kerry undergoes a laparoscopic cystectomy, and her pain settles with analgesia after 2 days. However, she is worried about ovarian cancer. What can you tell her, given she has the answer you gave in 4? **(1)**
7. Name two risk factors for ovarian cancer. **(2)**
8. What genetic mutations may increase the risk of ovarian cancer? **(1)**
9. Tumour markers can be used to monitor response to ovarian cancer treatment. Give an example of a tumour marker used in ovarian cancer. **(1)**

 **Q7** Poonam presents to your surgery with dysmenorrhoea. You are worried about endometriosis.

1. What is endometriosis? **(1)**
2. Name two sites where endometrial foci may commonly be found. **(2)**
3. Name a factor associated with endometriosis. **(1)**
4. Name two other symptoms found in endometriosis. **(2)**
5. What is the term used to describe endometrial glandular tissue found in the myometrium? **(1)**
6. Name two complications of endometriosis. **(2)**
7. Name two findings you may find on vaginal examination. **(2)**
8. Name two medical treatments for endometriosis. **(2)**
9. Name two possible surgical treatments for endometriosis. **(2)**

**Q8** Laura and Richard, both aged 30, come to see you, having spent a year trying to conceive, with no success. Neither partner has had children from previous relationships.

1. Explain the difference between primary and secondary infertility. **(1)**
2. Name three causes of female infertility. **(3)**
3. What lifestyle changes could you suggest? **(2)**
4. Name two blood tests to look at ovulatory function. **(2)**
5. Name one test to assess tubal patency. **(1)**
6. Laura's blood tests reveal anovulation and raised testosterone. On USS, there are multiple follicular cysts arranged in a pearl necklace fashion on each ovary. Name two possible symptoms of polycystic ovary syndrome (PCOS). **(2)**
7. Name two medical treatments to treat PCOS-associated infertility. **(2)**

**Q9** Natalie, aged 33, comes to see you about long-term contraception, as she has three children and feels she has finished her family.

1. List an advantage and a disadvantage of the following types of long-term contraception: laparoscopic tubal ligation; and hormone-releasing intrauterine contraceptive device. **(4)**
2. Natalie decides to undergo insertion of an IUCD. Name two contraindications to insertion. **(2)**
3. Natalie has an IUCD fitted. During the procedure, she feels faint and her heart rate is 40 bpm. What is the most likely explanation for this? **(1)**
4. Six days later, Natalie re-presents with acute lower abdominal pain, purulent vaginal discharge and a fever. What is the most likely diagnosis? **(1)**
5. Name two organisms that may be implicated in your answer above. **(2)**
6. How would you treat this disease initially? **(1)**
7. Name two possible complications of the disease you mentioned in 4. **(2)**

**Q10** Eleanor, aged 61, has been referred to gynaecology clinic on a 2-week-wait referral with post-menopausal bleeding. She is concerned about endometrial carcinoma.

1. Name two other causes of post-menopausal bleeding. **(2)**
2. What is the commonest histological type of endometrial carcinoma? **(1)**
3. Name two risk factors for endometrial carcinoma. **(2)**
4. Name the initial radiological investigation performed for post-menopausal bleeding. **(1)**
5. For stage I and II cancers, where tumour is confined to uterus and cervix, what is the recommended treatment? **(1)**
6. Name two treatments for higher-stage tumours. **(2)**
7. Name two sites where endometrial cancer metastasises to. **(2)**

# Elderly care

Q1  You are working nights as an FY1 and are called to see a 78-year-old lady who has fallen on the ward. She had woken up and was being walked to the bathroom by the staff nurse when she complained of feeling 'giddy', before slumping into the arms of the nurse. She appeared to lose consciousness for a few seconds. There was no head injury.

She had been admitted 2 days prior to the fall with pneumonia, for which she is receiving antibiotics. Her PMH includes hypertension, for which she takes ramipril, atenolol and bendroflumethiazide. You take a history of the fall and examine her fully. Of note, her blood pressure when lying down is 132/86, but it falls when she stands to 100/78. You suspect postural hypotension as the cause of her fall.

1. How is the diagnosis of postural hypotension made? **(1)**
2. What is the most likely cause of postural hypotension in this lady, given the above history? **(1)**
3. Give two other possible causes of postural hypotension. **(2)**
4. Give two non-pharmacological management options. **(2)**
5. Give two drugs that may be used to manage postural hypotension. **(2)**
6. Give two other factors that may increase the risk of falls in the elderly. **(2)**

**Q2** A 77-year-old man has been admitted to hospital by his GP with worsening confusion and a presumed UTI. He is unable to give any history and scores 1/10 on the AMTS. His daughter tells you that he hasn't been himself for the past week and is not normally confused. He lives alone, has no carers and is normally independent. He had previously been well and has not been started on any new medications. On examination, his temperature is 37.8°, HR 100 bpm reg, BP 116/74, RR 16 and O$_2$ sats 97% on air. His heart sounds are normal, chest is clear and his abdomen is soft, although he has some mild suprapubic tenderness. His urine is positive for nitrites and leucocytes.

1. Define delirium. **(2)**
2. What tool can be used to differentiate this from dementia? **(1)**
3. Other than infections, give three possible causes of delirium. **(3)**
4. Which organisms are most commonly responsible for UTIs? **(1)**
5. What is the mechanism of action of penicillin-based antibiotics? **(1)**
6. How may bacteria develop resistance to penicillin-based antibiotics? **(1)**

Many penicillin-based antibiotics are now used in combination with other drugs, for example, co-amoxiclav (amoxicillin + clavulanic acid) and tazocin (tazobactam + piperacillin).

7. How do these additional drugs work? **(1)**

 **Q3** An 84-year-old man is brought to his GP by his son, who is concerned regarding progressive memory loss. He is referred to a psychogeriatrician, who diagnoses Alzheimer's disease.

1. Other than memory loss, give two ways in which dementia may present. **(2)**
2. Give the two other commonest causes of dementia **(2)**
3. Give two common reversible causes of dementia. **(2)**
4. Name two abnormalities that may be seen on an MRI brain scan of a patient with Alzheimer's disease. **(2)**
5. What class of medication may be given to a patient with Alzheimer's disease? **(1)**
6. Briefly explain its mechanism of action. **(1)**

**Q4** A 72-year-old lady troubled by urinary incontinence visits her GP. She is a smoker and has developed a chronic cough. For the last few months, she reports passing a small amount of urine every time she coughs, and she is unable to control this. She believes the symptoms are worsening, and they are causing her significant distress. Her past medical history includes hypertension, for which she takes amlodipine, and COPD.

1. Which form of incontinence is she describing? **(1)**
2. Which group of muscles are commonly weak in women suffering with the above condition? **(1)**
3. Name one drug that may precipitate urinary incontinence. **(1)**
4. Give two reasons for weakness in these muscles. **(1)**
5. Name one drug that may cause urinary retention. **(1)**
6. Give two pieces of advice you would give her regarding how she could manage her condition conservatively. **(2)**
7. Duloxetine is a drug that is occasionally given to patients with incontinence. How does it help in these patients? **(2)**

The patient opts to manage her symptoms conservatively initially. She returns, reporting that her symptoms are again worsening. She has recently started a new tablet, as her blood pressure was found to be too high, despite being on amlodipine, and since then the symptoms have been worse.

8. What class of drug do you think may have been started? **(1)**

**5** A 73-year-old man is seen in A&E. He had experienced slurred speech and weakness on his left side. The symptoms lasted 50 minutes before resolving. On examination, he is in atrial fibrillation. You believe he may have had a TIA.

1. What scoring system can be used to determine the risk of stroke in the days following a transient ischaemic attack? **(1)**
2. Name three of the paramameters used in the scoring system above. **(3)**
3. What operation may be performed on someone with carotid artery stenosis? **(1)**
4. Name three risk factors for an ischaemic stroke. **(3)**

The same patient is seen in clinic soon after his attendance at A&E and is still in AF. He is started on warfarin.

5. What is the mechanism of action of warfarin? **(2)**

**6** A 77-year-old man is brought into A&E resus, having been found by his son slumped in his chair with facial droop and slurred speech. His son had seen him 4 hours previously, and he seemed well. Examination reveals an expressive dysphasia, right-sided facial palsy, right-sided weakness and right homonymous hemianopia. You suspect he has had a stroke, and an urgent CT scan reveals a large infarct in the middle cerebral artery territory.

1. From which artery does the middle cerebral artery arise? **(1)**
2. What is the name given to the arterial network in the brain? **(1)**
3. Using the Oxford Community Stroke Project (OCSP) classification, what is your diagnosis? **(3)**
4. What drug is commonly used for stroke thrombolysis? **(1)**
5. Give four absolute or relative contraindictaions to thrombolysis. **(4)**

**Q7** A 74-year-old lady has been brought into hospital by ambulance following recurrent falls at home. She has been seen by the doctors in A&E, who have diagnosed a fractured right pubic ramus, a common site for osteoporotic fractures, but they could find no cause for her recurrent falls. She has no carers at home and no close family, and an assessment by the occupational therapist in A&E has deemed it unsafe for her to go home on her own at this stage. She is taken to one of the medical wards for further assessment.

1. Give four risk factors for osteoporosis. **(2)**
2. Name three other sites where osteoporotic fragility fractures often occur. **(3)**
3. DEXA scanning is used to measure bone mineral density. What is meant by (a) T-score and (b) Z-score? **(2)**
4. She is started on 70 mg alendronate, a once-weekly bisphosphonate. Give two pieces of advice you would give her regarding how this should be taken. **(2)**
5. Give two common side effects of bisphosphonates. **(1)**

 **Q8** A 74-year-old man with known myeloma is admitted with severe back pain. He lives alone and has been taking paracetamol, but the pain has been gradually worsening over the past week. He had not visited his GP, as he was hoping the pain would settle down. His daughter visited today and brought him directly to A&E due to the pain he was in and weakness.

1. What two investigations are requested in a myeloma screen? **(2)**
2. What characteristic abnormality may be seen on plain radiographs of this myeloma? **(1)**

On direct questioning, he has been finding it difficult to pass urine and hasn't opened his bowels for 3 days. On examination, he has no sensation below T10.

3. What is your diagnosis? **(1)**
4. What drug should be started immediately? **(1)**
5. What urgent investigation would you request? **(1)**
6. Give two management options for this condition. **(2)**
7. Name two other possible complications of myeloma. **(2)**

**Q9** An 81-year-old man is referred to the neurology department by his GP. He has developed a tremor, and his GP is concerned he may have developed Parkinson's disease. The neurologist agrees and starts levodopa, in combination with benserazide (co-beneldopa/Madopar).

1. What is Parkinson's disease? **(1)**
2. Give the other two key features of Parkinson's disease. **(2)**
3. Name two other features of Parkinsonism. **(2)**
4. Name two other causes of Parkinsonism. **(2)**
5. Why is levodopa often used in combination with another drug, such as benserazide or carbidopa? **(1)**
6. Why is levodopa commonly not used in younger patients with Parkinson's disease? **(1)**

The next patient in the clinic is an 80-year-old man who also has a tremor. The tremor is worse when he is anxious, and affects his arms more than his legs. He has found that a small glass of whisky settles the tremor almost completely.

7. What is your diagnosis? **(1)**

**Q10** A 73-year-old man has been diagnosed with prostate cancer. He had seen his GP, complaining of nocturia, hesitancy and poor stream. His GP arranged a PSA, which was raised at 104, and TRUS biopsy, which confirmed prostate cancer. A subsequent bone scan revealed bony metastases in his spine and femur. He is deemed unfit for an operation, and instead managed with hormonal therapy. He is admitted to hospital with worsening confusion and abdominal pain. Blood tests on admission reveal a corrected calcium of 3.2 mmol/l.

1. Give two other causes of a raised PSA. **(2)**
2. What abnormality would you expect to see in his LFTs? **(1)**
3. Give two management options for his hypercalcaemia. **(2)**

He is discharged, but deteriorates over the following months. He becomes less independent and has carers to help him with toileting, washing, dressing and cooking. He is readmitted 6 months later with severe pneumonia. Despite an initial response to antibiotics, he deteriorates further, and your consultant decides to start the Liverpool Care Pathway (LCP).

4. Name the five distressing end-of-life symptoms that the LCP addresses, and name a drug it recommends to use for each. **(5)**

# Psychiatry

**Q1** Dawn, aged 37, is brought to the clinic by her concerned husband. He is worried that she has recently been staying out all night drinking alcohol (being previously teetotal), spending all of her wages and acting differently. You think this may be a manic episode.

1. List four symptoms associated with mania. **(4)**

Dawn tells you that she has 'a foolproof plan' at her local casino, and animatedly tells you about multiple affairs with other men.

2. Explain two possible detrimental social effects that acute mania can cause. **(2)**
3. List two possible medications, prescription or otherwise, that may be implicated in Dawn's symptoms. **(2)**
4. Dawn is eventually treated on an informal basis. What does being an informal patient mean? **(1)**
5. Dawn is started on long-term lithium. What 3 tests should be performed prior to treatment with lithium. **(3)**
6. Lithium can be dangerous in overdose. What must be considered before starting lithium? **(1)**
7. List two symptoms of lithium toxicity. **(1)**

Q2 Polly, aged 42, comes to your clinic about recurrently feeling low mood and loss of interest in playing squash or seeing friends for the last 3 weeks, with no precipitating event and no history of psychiatric disease.

1. What aspects of Polly's presentation may suggest depression? **(3)**
2. List four other symptoms of major depression that Polly may have. **(2)**
3. When dealing with a patient with depression, what important risk assessment must you undertake? **(1)**
4. You ask Polly to fill out a Hospital Anxiety and Depression Scale (HADS) score. Why are these scores useful in depression? **(2)**
5. What are the possible problems with HADS scores? **(2)**
6. List three possible treatments for this patient's depression. **(2)**
7. Depression may not occur in isolation. What other conditions may be associated with depression, which need to be screened for? **(2)**
8. Polly asks about the possibility of atypical depression. What difference is there between depression and atypical depression? **(1)**

Q3 You are asked to see Phyllis, an 87-year-old patient on an orthopaedic ward who has recently become very distressed and agitated. She is 3 days post-left hemiarthroplasty for a fractured neck of femur. She has a history of dementia, but her behaviour today is very different to how she is normally.

1. What is the difference between delirium and dementia? **(2)**
2. List four causes of delirium. **(2)**
3. List four causes of dementia. **(2)**
4. What non-medication treatment could you employ to help Phyllis? **(2)**
5. You decide to sedate Phyllis due to aggression and delirium. You prescribe her an IM dose of 5 mg haloperidol. What are the potential problems of using sedatives in the elderly and confused? **(2)**
6. Phyllis is treated with antibiotics for a hospital-acquired pneumonia and gradually improves. She lived at home prior to discharge. List four other healthcare professionals who can facilitate Phyllis's discharge. **(2)**
7. After discharge, Phyllis is referred to a psychiatrist specialising in the elderly. He performs a mini-mental state examination. Name two domains that a mental state examination should cover. **(1)**

**4** Steve, aged 39, goes to see his GP about a sore throat and during the consultation you notice he is slurring his words. On examination, he smells strongly of alcohol.

1. What are the recommended safe alcohol limits in units per day for men and women, according to the NHS? **(1)**
2. You find on further questioning that Steve drinks around 90 units per week. What is the definition of alcohol abuse? **(1)**
3. List 2 factors for Steve that might imply addiction. **(2)**
4. What treatments could you offer Steve in an effort to reduce drinking? **(2)**
5. Two weeks later, Steve attends the emergency department following a witnessed seizure, having not had enough money to buy a drink for 2 days. What are four other symptoms of alcohol withdrawal/delirium tremens? **(2)**
6. Having started Steve on chlordiazepoxide, he is also started on high-dose B and C vitamins (Pabrinex). Why has he been started on Pabrinex? **(1)**
7. Concerning long-term complications of alcohol abuse, name one example for the following systems: liver, CNS, CVS, GI tract. **(2)**
8. Steve is eventually started on Antabuse (disulfiram). How does this agent work in preventing relapse? **(1)**

**Q5** Samit, aged 20, is brought into hospital by the police, having been picked up in the city distressed and agitated and trying to break into a government building. He is very upset in A&E, claiming he was trying to stop the government from sending agents to capture him.

1. What risk factors are there for schizophrenia? **(2)**
2. What are the features of thought disorder in schizophrenia? **(1)**
3. Explain the following symptoms: thought broadcast, delusions, auditory hallucinations. **(3)**
4. List two negative symptoms of schizophrenia. **(1)**
5. During the interview, Samit becomes very agitated, he hyperventilates, starts shouting and clenches his fists over and over. What precautions should you take when interviewing potentially violent patients? **(1)**
6. Samit is admitted to the psychiatric unit under a section 3 and treated with an antipsychotic medication. Why are the following tests performed prior to initiation of treatment: fasting blood glucose, blood pressure, weight? **(2)**
7. Why can the use of antipsychotic medication cause hyperprolactinaemia? **(1)**
8. The day after starting on an antipsychotic, Samit develops some distressing restlessness, facial tics, slowed movement and a tremor. What drug reaction is being described? Explain the mechanism behind it. **(2)**
9. After having intolerance of two other antipsychotics, Samit is started on clozapine. Why does Samit need regular monitoring of full blood count whilst on this medication? **(1)**

**6** Claire, aged 23, is brought into hospital by the police on a section 136 following a domestic disturbance. She is well known to police and psychiatric services. Her symptoms include labile mood, black-and-white thinking, repeated self-harm and multiple unstable relationships. She has a diagnosis of personality disorder.

1. Which personality disorder is Claire likely to have? **(1)**
2. In order to be sectioned under the Mental Health Act, what must the patient be suffering from? **(1)**
3. What are the following sections of the Mental Health Act used for, and how long does each one last? Section 2, section 3, section 136. **(3)**
4. Why may Claire have a 'felt' stigma, as opposed to an 'enacted' stigma? **(2)**
5. Claire is admitted under a section 2 and does not want to be in hospital. How can she appeal against this? **(1)**
6. After leaving her section, Claire is brought into A&E following self-inflicted stab wounds. She is refusing all treatment. What must you assess in Claire for her to have 'capacity' to refuse treatment? **(3)**

**7** Jade, aged 18, is brought to see you by her concerned mother about her weight. She admits to losing weight intentionally and vomiting after eating.

1. Below which BMI level is a diagnosis of anorexia nervosa considered? **(1)**
2. What measures may patients take to achieve weight loss in this condition? **(2)**
3. Name two other mental illnesses that may coexist in Jade. **(2)**
4. What are two possible physical consequences of anorexia nervosa? **(2)**
5. How does bulimia nervosa differ from anorexia nervosa? **(1)**
6. Jade is admitted to an eating disorder unit. What is an advantage of treating patients in a unit as opposed to the community? **(2)**
7. Jade is commenced on a feeding programme to reverse her weight loss. Initially, her electrolytes are monitored. What is the reason for this? **(1)**

**Q8** Elizabeth, aged 27, has been brought into the emergency department by ambulance following an overdose.

1. List two factors that are important in the history of an overdose. **(2)**
2. If the patient presents within 1 hour of ingestion of a paracetamol overdose, name one treatment that is available. **(1)**
3. How does the treatment you listed in 2 work? **(1)**

A treatment nomogram comparing time from overdose to serum paracetamol level for the treatment of paracetamol overdose shows a normal treatment line and a high-risk treatment line. If the serum paracetamol level is above the treatment line, treatment should be started with N-acetylcysteine (NAC). A high-risk treatment line means a lower threshold to start treatment.

4. Name two factors that would put a patient on the high-risk treatment line. **(2)**
5. Elizabeth admits to taking 24 paracetamol 12 hours ago. Her plasma paracetamol at this time was 0.4 mmol/L. She was treated with NAC. Explain how NAC works in reducing liver damage. **(2)**
6. Following this treatment, name one blood test that should be performed regularly. **(1)**
7. Elisabeth is deemed medically fit for discharge after 48 hours. What other services may she benefit from before discharge? **(1)**
8. What are the gender differences with respect to suicide and deliberate self-harm? **(2)**
9. What are the worrying clinical features in DSH that would indicate high likelihood of a completed suicide in the future? **(2)**
10. How can you assess if somebody had suicidal intent for an episode of attempted suicide? **(1)**

**Q9** Jim, aged 34, comes to your GP clinic complaining of insomnia, abdominal pain and requesting that only morphine helps his symptoms. He is well known to drug and alcohol services locally for previous heroin use.

1. What clinical features may lead you to suspect drug use and drug-seeking behaviour? **(2)**
2. Jim admits to continued heroin use, has never tried to reduce his intake and has not thought about cutting down. What stage of the Prochaska and DiClemente transtheoretical model is Jim in? **(1)**
3. What advantages does using the transtheoretical model have in therapeutic intervention? **(1)**
4. What is a possible criticism of the transtheoretical model? **(1)**
5. Name four medical complications of prolonged heroin use. **(2)**
6. What detoxification programmes could be used in Jim's case when he is ready for an intervention? **(2)**
7. Three months after undergoing a detoxification programme, Jim is brought into A&E with reduced consciousness, having had a relapse. What are the initial steps in assessing this patient in A&E? **(1)**
8. What is the name of the drug used to treat acute opiate overdose? **(1)**
9. How would the onset and offset of action of the drug used in 8 affect your dosing? **(1)**

**Q10** Gillian, aged 37, comes to see you about 'her nerves', which she feels have been getting worse since her son has been abroad with the army. She fears she may be 'neurotic'.

1. What is the definition of neurosis? **(1)**
2. List four symptoms associated with anxiety. **(2)**
3. Gillian recently collapsed in the supermarket, thinking that she couldn't breathe with chest pain and palpitations. She was taken to hospital and no medical cause was found. What do you think happened to Gillian? **(1)**
4. How would cognitive behavioural therapy help Gillian? **(2)**
5. Gillian undergoes further treatment with relaxation therapy and graded exposure. Explain the term 'graded exposure'. **(1)**
6. You also decide to give Gillian a prescription for diazepam to help with anxiety. Why is this not a good long-term strategy? **(1)**
7. Name two other class of medications that may be used in Gillian's treatment. **(2)**
8. Gillian's son Damien comes to see you 6 months later, having just come back from abroad working for the army. He has been struggling since coming home. List three symptoms of post-traumatic stress disorder. **(2)**
9. What possible coping mechanisms should you ask Damien about? **(1)**

# Paediatrics

**Q1** An 8-month-old baby is brought to your GP surgery with a 2-day history of cough, audible wheeze and difficulty in breathing. Her birth was uneventful, and she has been well up until this point. You suspect this could be bronchiolitis.

1. Give four clinical signs that may be present on your examination. **(2)**
2. What is the commonest cause for this condition? **(1)**
3. What investigation can be performed to confirm the cause? **(1)**
4. What signs prompt admission? **(3)**
5. If the patient is to be admitted, what is involved in the treatment plan? **(2)**
6. If signs of severe bronchiolitis are present a chest X-ray would be performed. What would it be likely to show in bronchiolitis? **(1)**

**Q2** A 4-year-old girl attends the emergency department following a 3-day history of coughing and worsening difficulty in breathing, which both get worse at night. She has been well until now, apart from the odd episode of coryzal symptoms. Based on the history, you suspect croup.

1. How is the cough associated with croup usually described? **(1)**
2. What other symptoms, except for difficulty in breathing, are usually associated with this condition? **(2)**
3. Give two other causes of developing stridor in this age group. **(2)**
4. Name two viruses that are commonly responsible for causing croup. **(2)**
5. What treatment is typically prescribed? **(1)**
6. In severe disease, what else may be tried before escalation to intensive care? **(1)**
7. What are severe signs associated with croup? **(2)**

**Q3** A young child attends accident and emergency. His mother is very concerned that he has started vomiting after feeds. The vomiting is getting worse after feeds. He is still trying to feed and seems to be very hungry. You suspect congenital hypertrophic pyloric stenosis.

1. At what age does congenital hypertrophic pyloric stenosis usually present? **(1)**
2. Can bile be present as the condition progresses? Justify your answer. **(2)**
3. How is the vomiting after meals typically described? **(1)**
4. Where do you palpate to feel the pylorus in the abdomen during feeds? **(1)**
5. What acid-base disturbance would you expect to find? **(1)**
6. Name the four sections of the stomach. **(2)**
7. What two electrolyte abnormalities are associated with this condition? **(2)**

 **Q4** A young boy attends your GP clinic complaining of left-sided hip pain since yesterday. He is now limping due to pain in the hip on walking. He has also suffered with asthma, which is well controlled with salbutamol. You suspect a slipped upper femoral epiphysis (SUFE) after a full history and examination are concluded.

1. Which gender is more predisposed to SUFE? **(1)**
2. What age range is typical for this condition? **(1)**
3. Give two risk factors, other than gender, for a SUFE. **(2)**
4. What cartilage makes up the epiphyseal plate? **(1)**
5. What is typically found on examination? **(2)**
6. Name three differential diagnoses for hip pain in a child. **(3)**

Q5  A worried mother brings her newborn child into the GP practice, concerned that her baby is jaundiced. Regarding neonatal jaundice:

1. What is jaundice? **(2)**
2. Give two causes of jaundice within the first 24 hours of life. **(2)**
3. Give two investigations other than bilirubin levels which should be performed on a baby presenting with jaundice in the first 24 hours of life. **(2)**
4. What cause of prolonged jaundice should be suspected if the baby has pale stools and a raised conjugated bilirubin level? **(1)**
5. What complication may occur if raised levels of unconjugated bilirubin remain untreated? **(1)**
6. Give two methods of treating neonatal jaundice. **(2)**

Q6  A newborn is seen by the paediatric SHO for a routine baby check. On examination, a heart murmur is noted. Further investigation is undertaken, and the baby is found to have a congenital heart disease.

1. What prenatal investigation can be used to detect congenital heart diseases? **(1)**
2. In which direction is blood flowing in the heart in acyanotic congenital heart disease? **(1)**
3. Give two causes of acyanotic congenital heart disease. **(2)**
4. In which direction is blood flowing in the heart in cyanotic congenital heart disease? **(1)**
5. Give two causes of cyanotic congenital heart disease. **(2)**
6. In decompensated congenital heart disease, give two clinical features which may be seen. **(2)**
7. What is Eisenmenger's syndrome? **(1)**

**Q7** The paediatric resuscitation team is called to the maternity ward following delivery of a 26-week-old newborn with developed signs of infant respiratory distress syndrome (IRDS).

1. Apart from prematurity, give two risk factors for IRDS. **(2)**
2. What substance is deficient in the lungs of premature babies, giving rise to IRDS? **(1)**
3. What cells in the lungs produce this substance? **(1)**
4. What prenatal medication can be given to prevent respiratory distress syndrome? **(1)**
5. Give two signs of IRDS. **(2)**
6. What is seen on a chest X-ray in a baby with IRDS? **(1)**

Despite maximal therapy, the baby continues to deteriorate, and the resuscitation team recognises the baby is dying.

7. When breaking bad news, give two things a doctor can do to ensure a good consultation. **(2)**

 **Q8** A 2-year-old girl is brought to A&E after having a tonic-clonic seizure lasting 3 minutes. On further questioning, her parents report she has been unwell for the past few days and that she had felt hot immediately prior to the seizure. A febrile convulsion is suspected.

1. In what age range do febrile convulsions typically occur? **(1)**
2. Give two features that mean febrile seizures are classified as complex febrile convulsions. **(2)**
3. Give three investigations that should be considered. **(3)**
4. In a febrile seizure lasting more than 5 minutes, what class of drugs are first-line to attempt to stop the seizure? **(1)**
5. Give three bits of information to give the parents prior to the patient being discharged. **(3)**

**Q9** A 22-month-old boy is seen in the paediatric outpatients' clinic as his parents are concerned that he has not started walking. After further assessment, the child is diagnosed as having cerebral palsy.
1. Define cerebral palsy. **(2)**
2. Give two of the subtypes of cerebral palsy, using the classification system based on movement disorder. **(2)**
3. Apart from the motor complications, give two other clinical features that a child with cerebral palsy may have. **(2)**
4. Give two professional groups other than doctors that may be involved in the care of a child with cerebral palsy. **(2)**
5. Name two medications a child with cerebral palsy may be prescribed to help with muscle spasm. **(2)**

**Q10** A 9-month-old child is brought to A&E with crying, drawing up of the legs, vomiting and bloody red-currant jelly-like stools. Intussusception is suspected.
1. In which gender are intussusceptions more common? **(1)**
2. What may be found on abdominal palpation? **(1)**
3. Describe the pathogenesis occurring in intussusception. **(1)**
4. Give two possible findings on abdominal X-ray. **(2)**
5. Give two other investigations which may be performed. **(2)**
6. What non-surgical management option may be performed to avoid the need to take a patient to theatre? **(1)**
7. What are two indications for laparotomy? **(2)**

# Answers

# Cardiology

## A¹

1. Smoking, diabetes, hypertension, hypercholesterolaemia, +ve family history, male, increasing age, obesity, sedentary lifestyle. (½ a mark for each, max 2 marks)
2. Left anterior descending artery. (1)
3. Assess ABC, morphine, oxygen, GTN spray, 300 mg aspirin, contact cardiology/CCU/cath lab, LMWH. (1 mark for each, max 3 marks)
4. Primary PCI, thrombolysis. (1 mark for each, max 2 marks)
5. Aspirin, ACE inhibitor, β-blocker, statin, PRN GTN spray. (½ a mark for each, max 2 marks)

The major risk factors for ischaemic heart disease are smoking, hypertension, diabetes and hypercholesterolaemia. For the diagnosis of myocardial infarction, two of the following are required: cardiac-sounding chest pain, positive ECG changes and raised biochemical markers. If the ECG shows ST elevation, the diagnosis is an ST-segment elevation myocardial infarction (STEMI). If the cardiac enzymes are raised and the chest pain sounds cardiac, the diagnosis is a non-ST-segment elevation myocardial infarction (NSTEMI). Both are encompassed by the term acute coronary syndrome (ACS), as is unstable angina. This is angina of new onset, angina that is increasing in severity or frequency or angina that comes on with minimal exertion or at rest. Cardiac chest pain is often described as a crushing or heavy central pain and may radiate to the neck/jaw or arms. Many centres now offer 24-hour PCI, and this is the treatment of choice for the majority of patients. Following a myocardial infarction, patients should be taking aspirin, an ACE inhibitor, a β-blocker and a statin as long as there are no contraindications. In addition to these, clopidogrel should be taken for 1 year if PCI has been performed. Non-pharmacological measures also play a significant role, including cardiac rehabilitation programmes, smoking cessation, encouraging weight loss and dietary changes.

# A²

1. Leads I, aVL, V5 and V6. **(1)**
2. Left circumflex artery. **(1)**
3. Troponin (I/T), CK-MB, CK, AST, LDH. **(1 mark for each, max 2 marks)**
4. Inverted T waves, pathological Q waves. **(1 mark for each, max 2 marks)**
5. Not allowed to drive for 4 weeks, can drive from then on so long as not otherwise disqualified, DVLA do not need to be informed. **(1 mark for any of above points)**
6. Bleeding/haemorrhage, infection, MI, stroke, allergy to contrast, damage to coronary vessels requiring intervention, death. **(1 mark for each, max 3 marks)**

ECG changes tend to be seen in the leads that represent that territory of the myocardium, and each territory is supplied by a major coronary artery. The anterior leads are supplied by the left anterior descending artery and are represented by leads V1–V4. The lateral leads are supplied by the left circumflex artery and are represented by leads I, aVL, V5 and V6. The right coronary artery supplies the inferior myocardium, and this territory is represented by leads II, III and aVF. Immediate changes seen on an ECG following a STEMI are hyperacute T waves and then ST elevation (or new-onset left-bundle branch block). T-wave inversion and pathological Q waves develop over the next few days. Complications following an MI include cardiac arrest, arrhythmias, heart failure, DVT/ PE and pericarditis, among others.

# A³

1. Cold/windy weather, emotion (anger/excitement), lying down (decubitus angina), vivid dreams (nocturnal angina). **(1 mark for each, max 2 marks)**
2. Shortness of breath, sweating, feeling faint/light-headed. **(½ a mark for each, max 1 mark)**
3. FBC for anaemia, TFTs for thyrotoxicosis, lipid profile for hypercholesterolaemia, glucose (random/fasting/OGTT) for diabetes, U&Es for renal vessel disease/if considering ACEi **(½ a mark for each test, ½ a mark for each reason, max 2 named investigations, max 2 marks)**

4. ECG, exercise tolerance test (ETT)/exercise ECG, myocardial perfusion scintigraphy (MPS), echocardiography, coronary angiography. **(1 mark for each, max 3 marks)**

5. Irreversibly inhibits cyclooxygenase, which prevents further production of $TxA_2$ (thromboxine) from platelets as they do not have a nucleus, shifting the balance of $PGI_2 : TxA_2$ towards inhibiting platelet aggregation **(1 mark for each of above points, max 2 marks)**

Angina is central chest pain brought on by exercise and relieved by rest, and indicates coronary artery disease. Diagnosis is often made following the history, and there may be no obvious signs to find on examination, but you should look for signs of aortic stenosis, thyrotoxicosis and anaemia that would suggest the coronary arteries are not the problem. An ECG at rest is most likely to be normal, but signs of previous ischaemia, such as Q waves or left-bundle branch block, may be seen. Other investigations, such as exercise ECGs and myocardial perfusion scintigraphy, attempt to identify myocardial ischaemia following stress. Angiography may also be used to determine the coronary artery anatomy, and also if the diagnosis is unclear. Management should include identifying and managing risk factors for cardiovascular disease. A glyceryl trinitrate (GTN) spray may be used when the patient experiences chest pain. This is administered sublingually by the patient and causes coronary vasodilatation, hence improving blood flow through the arteries. Those with significant coronary artery disease often require percutaneous coronary intervention (PCI) or a coronary artery bypass graft (CABG), depending on the severity of their condition and the number of vessels involved.

## A4

1. Tachypnoea, tachycardia, raised JVP, fine lung crepitations, wheeze, additional heart sounds/gallop rhythm, dull percussion of bases, cyanosis, decreased tactile/vocal fremitus. **(1 mark for each, max 3 marks)**

2. FBC, U&Es, lipids, glucose, cardiac enzymes (troponin, CK-MB, LDH), ECG, chest X-ray, ABG, echocardiogram. **(½ a mark for each, max 2 marks)**

3. Furosemide, GTN/nitrates, morphine/diamorphine, oxygen. **(1 mark for each, max 2 marks)**

4. Furosemide. **(1)**
5. Orally (e.g. sando-K), IV (add KCl to IV fluids). **(2)**

Acute pulmonary oedema is a medical emergency. The patient should be sat up, as fluid accumulates at the lung bases, and given high-flow oxygen. IV furosemide is commonly given first-line to offload excess fluid. Morphine and nitrates are also used and act by reducing the preload. If these measures do not improve symptoms or if the patient remains hypotensive, inotropic support may be required, but an alternative diagnosis should also be considered. Many patients are treated for failure and infection simultaneously until a definitive diagnosis has been made. The causes of acute pulmonary oedema include post-MI, valvular disease and arrhythmias such as complete heart block. Non-cardiac causes include fluid overload (e.g. secondary to renal failure or a patient being given too much fluid intravenously), post-head injury and ARDS.

# A5

1. Inferior. **(1)**
2. Right coronary artery. **(1)**
3. Call for help/the crash team, start chest compressions. **(1 mark for each, max 2 marks)**
4. < 0.12 s (< 3 small squares). **(1)**
5. Normal QRS complex between VT complexes. **(1)**
6. Ventricular tachycardia. **(1)**
7. Yes – as no pulse palpable. **(1)**
8. Oxygen, adrenaline, amiodarone, lignocaine/lidocaine. **(1 mark for each, max 2 marks)**

A VT or VF cardiac arrest following a myocardial infarction is now seen less commonly, mainly due to the emergence of primary angioplasty. Distinguishing between VT and VF can be challenging, as both are seen on the ECG as tachycardia > 100 bpm, with broad QRS complexes (> 120 ms/> 3 small squares). The complexes seen in VF tend to appear more disorganised than those of VT, which appear regular and have complexes that appear more uniform. The commonest cause of broad complex tachycardia is VT, and if in doubt it should be managed as this. Immediate assessment of airway, breathing and circulation is vital, and high-flow oxygen should be given to all patients. If the patient is unresponsive and does not have a pulse, the arrest protocol should be followed. VF is a shockable rhythm. VT is a shockable rhythm if the patient does not have a palpable pulse. IV access should be obtained and bloods sent, particularly for $Mg^{2+}$ and $K^+$, as low levels of these can both predispose to VT/VF. Amiodarone and lignocaine (lidocaine) are both used to treat VT in a patient who is haemodynamically stable. In cases of recurrent VT, patients may be fitted with an implantable cardioverter-defibrillator (ICD), which detects the VT rhythm and delivers an immediate shock to the patient.

## A6

1.  New York Heart Association classification. **(1)**
2.  Dyspnoea, reduced exercise tolerance, fatigue, paroxysmal nocturnal dyspnoea (PND), orthopnoea, wheeze, cough (worse at night), pink, frothy sputum. **(1 mark for each, max 3 marks)**
3.  Alveolar/interstitial oedema in a 'bat's wings' distribution, Kerley B lines, cardiomegaly, upper lobe diversion, pleural effusions, fluid in the lung fissures. **(1 mark for each, max 3 marks)**
4.  Competitively inhibits the Na-K-2Cl cotransporter in the thick ascending limb of the loop of Henle, diminishing the osmotic gradient for water reabsorption. **(1 mark for action, 1 mark for site, max 2 marks)**
5.  Digoxin. **(1)**

Heart failure is an inability of the heart to provide an adequate cardiac output. Most commonly, this is due to low-output failure, for example, due to ischaemic heart disease, hypertension, valvular disease or heart block. In some cases, the body's requirements are high, for example, in those with thyrotoxicosis or Paget's disease, and even a higher than normal cardiac output is inadequate to meet the body's needs, causing symptoms. Symptoms of heart failure will depend on which ventricle is more affected. Left ventricular failure typically causes congestion in the pulmonary system, leading to dyspnoea, paroxysmal nocturnal dyspnoea (PND), orthopnoea and reduced exercise tolerance. Patients with right ventricular failure may complain of peripheral oedema, facial engorgement and distension of the abdomen. Congestive cardiac failure refers to heart failure affecting both ventricles, and patients with this will complain of symptoms of both. Patients with heart failure often have the characteristic ABCDE changes seen on their chest radiograph. Treatment includes treating any exacerbating factors, such as anaemia, addressing lifestyle factors, such as smoking, and pharmacological management with drugs such as diuretics, ACE inhibitors, β-blockers and digoxin.

# A7

1. 32.5 (weight (kg)/height (m)$^2$). **(1)**
2. Obese. **(1)**
3. Aim to lose weight, stop smoking, low-fat diet, low salt intake, increase exercise, reduce alcohol intake. **(1 mark for each, max 3 marks)**
4. ACE inhibitor. **(1)**
5. Hypotension (particularly first-dose hypertension), dry cough, renal impairment, hyperkalaema, angioedema/urticaria. **(1 mark for each, max 2 marks)**
6. Silver/copper wiring, A-V nipping, flame haemorrhages, cotton wool spots, papilloedema. **(1 mark for each, max 2 marks)**

Hypertension is a major risk factor for ischaemic heart disease, stroke, chronic kidney disease, heart failure and many more. Deciding when to start treatment for this can be difficult. Current guidelines suggest starting treatment on all patients with a sustained blood pressure ≥ 160/100 mmHg. In patients whose blood pressure is not quite this high, but is ≥ 140/90, other cardiac risk factors should be assessed and a decision made in conjunction with the patient regarding whether to start antihypertensive medication. ACE inhibitors are first-line drugs in those < 55 who are not of Afro-Carribean descent. Those of Afro-Carribean descent or those > 55 are now treated with a calcium channel blocker (CCB) first-line. NICE guidelines regarding hypertension were changed slightly in August 2011. Previously, guidelines stated that a CCB or a thiazide diuretic could be used first-line in those of Afro-Carribean descent or in those > 55. Diuretics are no longer first-line, although they should be used if there are contraindications to starting a CCB. Also, the diuretic of choice was previously a thiazide diuretic, such as bendroflumethiazide. This has now changed to a thiazide-like diuretic, such as indapamide or chlortalidone. Patients already established on a thiazide diuretic and whose hypertension is well controlled should continue this.

# A⁸

1. Calcium channel blocker. **(1)**
2. Heart failure, ischaemic heart disease, stroke, chronic kidney disease (hypertensive nephropathy), hypertensive retinopathy, aneurysmal disease, peripheral vascular disease. **(1 mark for each, max 3 marks)**
3. Inhibits HMG-CoA reductase, the rate-limiting step in cholesterol synthesis. **(1 mark for enzyme, 1 mark for cholesterol synthesis)**
4. Xanthelasmata, tendon xanthoma, corneal arcus, other xanthomatas (eruptive, tuberous, palmar). **(1 mark for each, max 2 marks)**
5. Gout. **(1)**
6. NSAID (e.g. indomethacin, ibuprofen, diclofenac, naproxen), colchicines. **(1 mark for any of above)**

Both hypertension and hypercholesterolaemia are risk factors for cardio-vascular disease. Statins are commonly used to lower cholesterol levels in patients whose levels are too high, following an MI and in those that are at high risk of cardiovascular disease. The West of Scotland Coronary Prevention Trial found that taking a statin daily reduces the incidence of primary cardiac events in those with no signs of cardiac disease by up to one third. The Heart Protection Study later found that those known to be high risk for developing cardiac disease but have normal cholesterol also benefit from taking statins. They are generally well tolerated, although some patients complain of muscular aches and pains, particularly of the legs. The main side effect of concern is reversible myositis, which causes severe muscle pains, a raised creatinine kinase (CK) and may lead to rhabdomyolysis.

# A⁹

1. Atrial fibrillation. **(1)**
2. Pneumonia, myocardial infarction, pulmonary embolism, hyperthyroidism, alcohol excess, heart failure, endocarditis. **(1 mark for each, max 3 marks)**
3. Irregular QRS complexes, absence of P waves. **(1 mark for each, max 2 marks)**
4. Shortness of breath, light-headedness/dizziness/syncope, chest pain. **(½ a mark for each, max 1 mark)**

5. Medical (e.g. amiodarone, flecainide), electrical (e.g. DC cardioversion), ablation. **(1 mark for each, max 2 marks)**
6. β-blocker, calcium channel blocker, digoxin, warfarin. **(½ a mark for each, max 1 mark)**
7. Stroke, transient ischaemic attack (TIA), heart failure, systemic emboli, falls. **(½ a mark for each, max 1 mark)**

Atrial fibrillation is fast irregular atrial rhythm whereby the atria discharge electrical current between 300 to 600 times per minute. The origin of the impulses is the pulmonary veins or atria themselves. The atrioventricular node only responds intermittently to this, which gives the irregular rhythm. It has a large variety of causes. The mainstay of treatment is to treat the underlying cause and to try and revert the heart rhythm back to sinus. This can be done through using either medication, electrical current or ablation. When treating the patient, it is also important to be aware of the complications, the most important being stroke. To prevent this, anticoagulation is required. The $CHADS_2$ score can be used to help the physician decide between aspirin or warfarin as a suitable anticoagulant.

# A10

1. Assess airway, breathing and circulation, correcting abnormalities at each stage. **(3)**
2. Viridans streptococci. **(1)**
3. Microscopic haematuria. **(1)**
4. Roth spot. **(1)**
5. Duke criteria. **(1)**
6. Collapsing pulse, wide pulse pressure, displaced apex beat, Duroziez's sign (femoral diastolic murmur), Quincke's sign (nail-bed capillary pulsation), Traube's sign/pistol shot femorals ('pistol shot' sound over femoral arteries), Corrigan's sign (carotid pulsation), de Musset's sign (head nodding), Austin Flint murmur (mid-diastolic murmur heard in severe aortic regurge due to fluttering of the anterior mitral cusp). **(1 mark for each, max 3 marks)**

Infective endocarditis must be suspected in anyone with a fever and a new murmur. This condition often takes a subacute course, and common presenting symptoms include fever, rigors, night sweats, dyspnoea and general malaise. If this is suspected, the case should be discussed early with a cardiologist and microbiologist to ensure prompt and appropriate treatment. As well as listening to heart sounds to identify the affected valve, examination should include inspection of the hands for clubbing, splinter haemorrhages, Osler's nodes and Janeway lesions. Also examine the fundi, looking for Roth spots, and dip the urine, looking for microscopic haematuria. Blood tests typically show a raised WCC and inflammatory markers. All patients should have echocardiography performed at the earliest opportunity. The Duke criteria are used to make this diagnosis, and require two major + one minor criteria, or one major and three minor criteria, or all five minor criteria. The major criteria are positive blood cultures and evidence of endocarditis seen on echocardiography. The minor criteria are a known predisposition to endocarditis, fever > 38°, vascular/immunological signs on examination, positive blood cultures not meeting major criteria and echocardiography findings which may be compatible with endocarditis but do not meet the major criteria. Treatment is commonly with relatively long courses of antibiotics. Occasionally, surgical intervention may be required.

## A¹¹

1. Tricuspid regurgitation. **(1)**
2. *Staphylococcus aureus.* **(1)**
3. Three sets, from different sites, three different times. **(1 mark for each, max 3 marks)**
4. Chest X-ray, echocardiogram, ECG, urine dip. **(1 mark for each, max 2 marks)**
5. Prosthetic valves, patent ductus arteriosis, VSD, coarctation, mitral valve disease, aortic valve disease (e.g. bicuspid aortic valve). **(1 mark for each, max 2 marks)**
6. Prophylactic antibiotics prior to invasive procedures. **(1)**

Many patients have a predisposition to developing endocarditis. Valvular lesions, such as a bicuspid aortic valve, a ventricular septal defect (VSD) or patent ductus arteriosus (PDA), all carry an increased risk of developing this condition. In these patients, the infection is commonly seen on valves on the left side of the heart. Viridans streptococci are the commonest causative organism, but enterococci, *S. aureus* and the HACEK group (*Haemophilus, Actinobacillus, Cardiobacterium, Eikenella, Kingella*) may also be responsible. Intravenous drug users (IVDUs) are also at increased risk of developing endocarditis, as they often inadvertently introduce organisms directly into the venous system. Endocarditis in these patients commonly affects valves on the right side of the heart, and is usually caused by *S. aureus*. Three sets of blood cultures should be taken from three different sites at three different times and at peak fever in order to identify the causative organism.

# Respiratory

## A¹

1. House dust mite, pollen, domestic pets, cold air, exercise, emotion, infection, cigarette smoke, drugs (e.g. NSAIDs, β-blockers). **(1 mark for each, max 4 marks)**
2. Obstructive pattern (reduced $FEV_1$ : FVC ratio). **(1)**
3. Improvement in $FEV_1$ by > 15% following administration of bronchodilator. **(1)**
4. Long-acting β-agonist, e.g. salmeterol **(1)**
5. Eczema, allergic rhinitis/hay fever, food allergies/intolerance/anaphylaxis, contact dermatitis (e.g. latex allergy), urticaria. **(1 mark for each, max 2 marks)**
6. Stimulates β2 receptors of respiratory tract, which increases sympathetic activity and relaxes bronchial smooth muscle. **(1)**

Asthma commonly presents in childhood and is characterised by reversible airway obstruction, hyperresponsiveness of the airways to numerous allergens and inflammation of the bronchi. Symptoms tend to be wheeze, dry cough, shortness of breath and chest tightness. Childhood asthma is commonly associated with other atopic conditions, such as hay fever and eczema, and most cases resolve by adulthood. Common triggers include viral infections, exercise, cold air, the house dust mite and pollen. NSAIDs also trigger asthma in 5%–10% of patients with asthma, so it is important to use these with caution in patients who have not received them before. Treatment is initially with inhaled salbutamol as required, and the British Thoracic Society have step-wise management guidelines for further treatment if this is not sufficient, and information on when referral to secondary care is advised.

## A²

1. 72 (20 per day for 1 year = 1 pack-year; 30 per day = 1.5 pack-years, $1.5 \times 48 = 72$). **(1)**
2. Obstructive. **(1)**
3. $FEV_1$. **(1)**

4. Type 2 respiratory failure, respiratory acidosis. **(1 mark for each, max 2 marks)**

5. Requires controlled oxygen therapy via venturi mask as is at risk of losing hypoxic drive. **(1 mark for implication, 1 mark for reason, max 2 marks)**

6. Antibiotics, steroids, salbutamol/ipratropium nebulisers, chest physiotherapy, consider non-invasive ventilation (NIV) (e.g. BiPAP, CPAP), repeat blood gases, inform senior colleagues. **(1 mark for each, max 2 marks)**

7. He continues to smoke. **(1)**

COPD is an irreversible, often progressive disease characterised by airway obstruction that is not fully reversible. The term COPD encompasses chronic bronchitis and emphysema. The major risk factor for the development of COPD is smoking tobacco, but it is also seen in coal miners. Patients commonly present with a chronic productive cough, shortness of breath and wheeze. Lung function testing reveals an obstructive pattern with little or no reversibility. Infective exacerbations of COPD are common and managed with bronchodilators, steroids and antibiotics, as well as chest physiotherapy to help remove retained secretions. Controlled oxygen therapy in these patients is important. If their blood gas reveals a high $pCO_2$ and low $pO_2$ they are reliant upon their hypoxic drive to maintain ventilation. Large concentrations of oxygen will increase their $pO_2$ but reduce their respiratory drive, hence raising the $pCO_2$ and worsening the respiratory failure and respiratory acidosis. Oxygen should be administered via a venturi mask, initially at 24%. Ventilatory support may be required if there is a rising $pCO_2$ or falling pH, hence it is important to monitor the blood gases in these patients regularly.

# A³

1. Reduced chest expansion, dull percussion note, increased tactile vocal fremitus, increased vocal resonance, bronchial breathing. **(1 mark for each, max 2 marks)**

2. CXR, ABG, sputum culture, urine pneumococcal antigen. **(1 mark for each, max 2 marks)**

3. Two – scores for age (> 65) and urea (> 7). **(1 mark for correct score, 1 mark for reasoning, max 2 marks)**

4. *S. pneumoniae, Haemophilus influenzae, Mycoplasma pneumoniae.*
   **(1 mark for each, max 3 marks)**
5. Stop simvastatin – increased risk of myositis. **(1)**

Pneumonia is an infection of the lung parenchyma. Patients commonly present with fever, worsening dyspnoea and a productive cough. It can be particularly severe in elderly patients, and is a common cause of death in this group. Pneumonia can be classified in numerous ways. Community-acquired pneumonia is commonly caused by *S. pneumoniae, H. influenzae* and *M. pneumoniae.* Atypical agents include *Legionella pneumophila* and *S. aureus,* among others. Hospital acquired/nosocomial pneumonia is defined as pneumonia that develops within 48 hours of hospital admission, and is often more severe due to antibiotic resistance. Gram-negative bacilli are often responsible, as is *Pseudomonas aeruginosa.* The CURB-65 score is used to determine the severity of community-acquired pneumonia and determine whether the patient is safe to be treated in the community or requires hospital admission. Antibiotics, IV fluids and oxygen, if necessary, are the mainstays of treatment.

## A4

1. Abbreviated mental test score (AMTS), urea, respiratory rate, blood pressure. **(1 mark for each, max 4 marks)**
2. Will need hospital treatment because patients with a CURB-65 score of > 1 require hospital admission. **(1)**
3. Pleural effusion, respiratory failure, empyema, lung abscess, septicaemia, AF, shock, pericarditis/myocarditis, cholestatic jaundice. **(1 mark for each, max 2 marks)**
4.

|  | Chest expansion | Percussion note | Auscultation |
|---|---|---|---|
| **Consolidation** | Reduced | Dull | Bronchial breathing/ crepitations |
| **Pleural effusion** | Reduced | Stony dull | Diminished breath sounds |
| **Pneumothorax** | Reduced | Hyperresonant | Diminished breath sounds |

**(1 mark per chest problem, all 3 signs required for 1 mark, max 3 marks)**

Antibiotics are often started empirically according to local protocols until the results of blood and sputum cultures are available. If a patient is failing to respond to antibiotics and there are no sensitivities available, it is often appropriate to discuss the case with a microbiologist, who may suggest an alternative drug. Consolidation of the lung, or specific lobe, is seen as increased opacification of the lung fields in that distribution on the chest X-ray. This may take several weeks to return to normal, despite treatment with appropriate antibiotics and clinical improvement, so a repeat chest X-ray is often recommended at 6 weeks to ensure this. The differential diagnosis of acute pleuritic chest pain includes pneumonia, pulmonary embolism and pneumothorax. The majority of pneumothoraces can be excluded on a plain chest radiograph, but diagnosing a PE is often more difficult, even if there are signs of pneumonia on examination and on the chest X-ray. For this reason, patients are often treated for both conditions simultaneously until a definitive diagnosis has been established.

# A5

1. HIV/AIDS prevalence, use of immunosuppressive drugs, poor socio-economic conditions and overcrowding, increased immigration from areas of high prevalence of TB, multidrug resistance. **(1 mark for each, max 2 marks)**
2. Rifampicin (6 months), isoniazid (6 months), pyrazinamide (2 months), ethambutol (2 months). **(½ a mark for drug, ½ a mark for length of course, max 4 marks)**
3. To combat multidrug resistance. **(1)**
4. Side effect of rifampicin. **(1)**
5. Erythema nodosum. **(1)**
6. Idiopathic, Crohn's disease, ulcerative colitis, sarcoidosis, drugs (e.g. oral contraceptive, sulphonamides), streptococcal infection, chlamydia, leprosy. **(1 mark for each, max 2 marks)**

The number of cases of TB worldwide has risen rapidly due to increased immunosuppression (from HIV/AIDS and immunosuppressive drugs), increased immigration from endemic areas, the emergence of multidrug-resistant forms of TB and reduced socio-economic conditions. Primary tuberculosis is the first infection with the organism. It is usually asymptomatic, but may cause cough, wheeze and erythema nodosum. In most cases, the primary infection resolves and the patient remains well until reactivation of the organism occurs years later due to malnutrition or immunosuppression, and post-primary TB occurs. Occasionally, the primary infection progresses, leading to more widespread disease. Miliary TB refers to dissemination of the organism via the bloodstream and is fatal without treatment. TB can also affect many other parts of the body, such as the eyes, skin, lymph nodes, bones/joints and CNS, such as TB meningitis. Treatment is with multiple antibiotics to combat multidrug resistance, and is for 6 months in cases of pulmonary TB, 9 months for TB affecting bone and 12 months for TB meningitis. A low index of suspicion should be held for TB in any areas where the disease is prevalent.

## A⁶

1. One in 2500 live births. **(1)**
2. Chronic infection of the large airways, causing their abnormal, permanent dilatation. **(2)**
3. *S. pneumoniae, H. influenzae, P. aeruginosa, Burkholderia cepacia* **(1 mark for each, max 2 marks)**
4. Idiopathic, post-infective (inadequately or non-treated necrotising infections, e.g. *S. aureus*, *Mycoplasma pneumoniae*, pertussis, measles, TB, *Klebsiella* sp), post-obstructive (foreign body, tumour, hilar lymphadenopathy, broncholithiasis), congenital (Young's syndrome, primary ciliary dyskinesia, Kartagener's syndrome), immunodeficiency, allergic bronchopulmonary aspergillosis, α1-antitrypsin deficiency, rheumatoid arthritis, ulcerative colitis. **(1 mark for each, max 3 marks)**
5. Pneumonia, septicaemia, recurrent pneumonia/LRTIs, haemoptysis, respiratory failure, cor pulmonale, pneumothorax. **(1 mark for each, max 2 marks)**

Bronchiectasis is abnormal, permanent dilatation of the bronchi and bronchioles caused by chronic infection of these airways. The ability to clear secretions from the respiratory tract is therefore impaired, hence patients present with a chronic productive cough. Other symptoms include occasional haemoptysis and recurrent respiratory tract infections. Examination signs include clubbing of the fingernails and coarse crepitations on auscultation of the chest. High-resolution CT scanning of the chest is the investigation of choice to confirm the diagnosis. Management includes chest physiotherapy, antibiotics guided by the results of cultures and sensitivities, and bronchodilators. Massive haemoptysis may occur due to the high pressure in the bronchial arteries, and this is fatal in 25% of cases. The majority of cases settle with rest, antibiotics and blood transfusion, but some cases may require embolisation of the culprit vessel or surgical resection.

# A⁷

1. Known malignancy, immobility, pregnancy, COCP/HRT, thrombophillia, known DVT, previous DVT/PE, family history DVT/PE, major trauma, inflammatory disease, nephrotic syndrome, dehydration, current infection. **(1 mark for each, max 2 marks)**
2. Type 1 respiratory failure **(1)**
3. Ventilation/perfusion mismatch. **(1)**
4. VQ scan, CTPA. **(1 mark for each, max 2 marks)**
5. 2–3. **(1)**
6. 6 months. **(1)**
7. Prophylactic LMWH, TED stockings, early mobilisation, intermittent pneumatic compression devices. **(1 mark for each, max 2 marks)**

Pulmonary emboli arise from thrombus that forms in the venous system, commonly in the legs or pelvis. Part of the thrombus dislodges and embolises through the right side of the heart into the pulmonary arteries. Patients commonly present with dyspnoea, but may also complain of pleuritic chest pain and occasionally haemoptysis. Massive emboli may cause collapse and sudden death. The classical ECG changes associated with a PE are deep S waves in lead I, pathological Q waves in lead III and inverted T waves in lead III ($S_IQ_{III}T_{III}$), although this is rarely seen. A sinus tachycardia is the commonest finding, but it is important to look for signs of right ventricular strain. A CTPA is the most commonly used investigation to diagnose PEs, and the emboli appear as filling defects as contrast flows through the pulmonary arteries. A V/Q scan is an alternative. Treatment is usually with anticoagulation. Warfarin is most commonly used, and the target INR is 2–3. A low molecular weight heparin (LMWH), such as dalteparin or tinzaparin, is used until this is in the desired range. Patients are treated for 6 months if this is their first DVT or PE. If they have a previous history of DVT/PE, then warfarin is continued lifelong. Major risk factors for thromboembolic disease include malignancy, recent major surgery and immobility. Some medical conditions predispose to the formation of venous thrombus, such as antiphospholipid syndrome and thrombophilia.

## A⁸

1. Cough, haemoptysis, dyspnoea, chest pain, hoarse voice, weight loss, anorexia, Horner's syndrome. (½ **a mark for each, max 2 marks**)
2. Brain, bone, liver, lung (other sites), adrenals. (**1 mark for each, max 3 marks**)
3. CT, PET scan, bone scan. (**1 mark for each, max 2 marks**)
4. TNM. (**1**)
5. Superior vena caval obstruction. (**1**)
6. Pemberton's test. (**1**)

Lung cancer presents in a number of ways. The commonest presentation is an unresolving cough in a smoker, but it may be detected on routine chest X-ray in a patient without symptoms. Smoking is the major risk factor for the development of lung cancer. Lung cancers are subcategorised as small cell lung cancer and non-small cell lung cancer. This differentiation is important, as it has implications regarding the prognosis, staging and treatment of the cancer. Non-small cell lung cancer is further subdivided, and the commonest forms are squamous cell carcinoma, adenocarcinoma and large cell carcinoma. TNM staging is used for non-small cell cancer, and the treatment of choice for low-grade disease is surgical excision. Curative radiotherapy is an alternative. Small cell lung cancer is staged as limited or extensive disease. The disease carries a poor prognosis, but may be responsive to chemotherapy.

## A⁹

1. Reduced lung volume, reticulonodular shadowing (often worse in lower zones), honeycomb lung (advanced disease). (**1 mark for each, max 2 marks**)
2. Answers: (a) low; (b) low; (c) high/normal. (**1 mark for each, max 3 marks**)
3. Farmer's lung, bird fancier's lung, maltworker's lung, humidifier fever, mushroom worker's lung, cheese washer's lung, winemaker's lung. (**1 mark for each, max 2 marks**)

4. Systemic sclerosis, rheumatoid arthritis, drugs (e.g. bleomycin, amiodarone, nitrofurantoin, methotrexate), SLE, Sjögren's syndrome, ulcerative colitis, tuberous sclerosis, neurofibromatosis. (½ a mark for each, max 1 mark)

5. Bronchial carcinoma, mesothelioma, bronchiectasis, cryptogenic organising pneumonia, chronic empyema, chronic lung abscess. (1 mark for each, max 2 marks)

Interstitial lung disease is a term that encompasses a large number of disorders that cause diffuse disease of the lung parenchyma. Spirometry of patients with ILD shows a restrictive pattern, and the classical chest X-ray appearance of 'honeycomb lung' occurs in severe cases. Extrinsic allergic alveolitis occurs secondary to inhalation of allergens that causes a hypersensitivity reaction within the lungs. This commonly causes an acute illness in which the patient develops fever, shortness of breath and a dry cough 4–6 hours following exposure to the allergen. Repeated exposure over time can lead to chronic disease in which the patient complains of chronic dry cough, worsening dyspnoea, reduced exercise tolerance and weight loss. Prevention of exposure to the allergen in patients known to have the condition is the key management strategy. Causes of extrinsic allergic alveolitis include farmer's lung and bird fancier's lung. Interstitial lung disease may also be secondary to known medical conditions, such as rheumatoid arthritis or systemic sclerosis, or certain medications, such as amiodarone or nitrofurantoin. Often, however, no cause is found and the patient is diagnosed with idiopathic pulmonary fibrosis. The prognosis of this is poor, and mortality in the acute form is high.

## A¹⁰

1. Obstructive sleep apnoea. (1)
2. Epworth sleepiness scale/score. (1)
3. Acromegaly, enlarged tonsils, enlarged adenoids, nasal polyps, alcohol. (1 mark for each, max 2 marks)
4. Sleep studies. (1)
5. Weight loss, avoid alcohol, sleep upright, mandibular advancement device, CPAP, surgery (e.g. adenoidectomy etc.). (1 mark for each, max 2 marks)
6. Right heart failure secondary to chronic pulmonary hypertension. (1)

7. Dilatation right atrium, enlarged right ventricle, prominent pulmonary arteries. **(1 mark for each, max 1 mark)**
8. Right axis deviation, P pulmonale, dominant R wave in V1, inverted T waves in the chest leads. **(1 mark for each, max 1 mark)**

Classically, obstructive sleep apnoea affects overweight, middle-aged men. It is often their partner that is most concerned, as they witness the apnoeic episodes. They often give a long history of snoring, but may complain of feeling increasingly tired, or falling asleep, during the day. Relaxation of the muscles responsible for maintaining the airway during sleep causes occlusion of the airway, resulting in apnoeic episodes. Each time this happens, the patient is woken from sleep due to hypoxia. This may happen hundreds of times per night, but occurs for such a short period of time they are unaware of it. The Epworth Sleepiness Scale is a questionnaire that helps determine the degree of sleepiness during the day, asking the likelihood that the patient would fall asleep in a number of everyday scenarios. Sleep studies are ultimately used to confirm the diagnosis, requiring evidence of at least 15 apnoeic/hypopnoeic episodes per hour of sleep. Simple management strategies include sleeping more upright, losing weight and avoiding alcohol/tobacco. If these fail, CPAP increases the pressure in the pharynx, helping to maintain the airway during sleep. This, however, is poorly tolerated in a number of patients.

## A¹¹

1. Lymphoma, bronchial carcinoma, TB, *Mycoplasma*, extrinsic allergic alveolitis. **(1 mark for each, max 2 marks)**
2. Non-caseating granulomas. **(1)**
3. Skin (erythema nodosum), ocular (anterior uveitis, posterior uveitis, keratoconjunctivitis sicca), musculoskeletal (arthralgia, bone cysts), CNS (neuropathy, cranial nerve palsies), cardiac (cardiomyopathy, ventricular dysrhythmias), other (lymphadenopathy, hepatosplenomegaly, hypercalcaemia). **(½ a mark for each, max 2 marks)**
4. Do not stop taking steroids suddenly, doses should only be reduced gradually, carry 'steroid card' at all times, doses need to be increased at times of intercurrent illness, always inform doctors and dentists prior to treatment/surgery, inform of side effects. **(1 mark for each, max 2 marks)**

5. Endocrine (adrenal suppression, hyperglycaemia), change in fat distribution (central obesity, buffalo hump, moon face), skin (bruising, skin thinning), eyes (cataracts), musculoskeletal (muscle wasting, osteoporosis, avascular necrosis of the femoral head), psychosis, euphoria, emotional liability, CVS (hypertension), other (increased susceptibility to infection, peptic ulceration) (½ a mark for each, max 3 marks)

Sarcoidosis is a multisystem granulomatous condition of unknown aetiology. It is often diagnosed following a routine chest X-ray which has revealed bilateral hilar lymphadenopathy. It commonly affects the lungs, causing worsening pulmonary fibrosis, and in severe cares cor pulmonale and death. Extrapulmonary features are seen in many patients and may include disease of the skin, eyes and joints. Other investigations of use are transbronchial biopsy (to identify non-caseating granulomas), serum ACE (which is raised) and lung function tests (which reveal a restrictive pattern due to the fibrosis and are used to monitor disease progression). Corticosteroids are the mainstay of treatment. Of those with hilar lymphadenopathy alone, two thirds of cases resolve spontaneously within 2 years.

# A¹²

1. Reduced chest expansion on the affected side, dull percussion note, reduced tactile vocal fremitus, reduced/absent breath sounds, reduced vocal resonance, tracheal deviation away from the effusion if large. (1 mark for each, max 2 marks)
2. Above the rib, to avoid the neurovascular bundle that is located immediately beneath the ribs. (1 mark for correct site, 1 mark for reason, max 2 marks)
3. Exudate. (1)
4. Exudate. (1)
5. Microscopy, culture and sensitivities, cytology, glucose, amylase, pH, Ziehl-Neelsen staining for acid-fast bacilli. (1 mark for each, max 2 marks)
6. Pleurodesis with talc, bleomycin, tetracycline. (1 mark for procedure, 1 mark for chemical, max 2 marks)

Fluid in the pleural space is known as a pleural effusion. The fluid may be a transudate or an exudate. Transudates are commonly caused by cardiac failure, cirrhosis or renal failure. Exudates have high protein content and are commonly due to infection, inflammation or malignancy. Examination of the chest classically reveals reduced chest expansion on that side, a 'stony dull' percussion note and reduced breath sounds. Small effusions may be seen on a chest X-ray as blunting of the costophrenic angle. Larger effusions are seen more clearly as a fluid level/meniscus in the lung fields. A diagnostic aspiration is performed to determine the nature of the effusion. Drainage may be required if the effusion is causing symptoms. If pleural effusions are recurrent, pleurodesis may be necessary. This involves the installation of an irritant, such as talc, into the pleural space to cause local inflammation and fusion of the pleura to the chest wall. Persistent collections may require surgical intervention.

# Renal

## A¹

1.  Stage 3. **(1)**
2.  Hypertension, glomerulonephritis, renovascular disease, pyelonephritis, polycystic kidney disease, obstructive uropathy. **(½ a mark for each, max 2 marks)**
3.  Exclude obstruction, assess renal size, exclude polycystic kidneys. **(1 mark for each, max 2 marks)**
4.  ACE inhibitor. **(1)**
5.  Dry cough, first-dose hypotension, hyperkalaemia, acute renal failure, urticaria. **(1 mark for each, max 2 marks)**
6.  $Ca^{2+}$, $PO_4^{3-}$, alk phos, PTH, FBC. **(1 mark for each, max 2 marks)**

Chronic kidney disease (CKD) is classified, according to the eGFR, into five stages. Patients are usually asymptomatic until stage 4, i.e. eGFR 15–29 mL/min. The commonest causes of CKD are diabetes, hypertension, renovascular disease and glomerulonephritis. Investigations are performed to rule out reversible causes of CKD, such as obstruction of the renal tract, but often there is very little that can be done to reverse the disease progress. Measures can be taken, however, to halt the disease progression. Measures include treating hypertension and other cardiac risk factors. ACE inhibitors have also been shown to be beneficial in those with CKD and proteinuria, and patients should be warned of potential side effects prior to starting them. Complications, such as anaemia and renal osteodystrophy, should also be managed appropriately. Patients with CKD often require lower doses of drugs that are excreted renally to prevent accumulation of the drug and toxicity. Examples of these include gentamicin and digoxin. Patients with CKD are prone to developing hyperkalaemia, and a low-potassium diet is advised for all patients.

## A²

1.  Stage 5. **(1)**
2.  Pallor, uraemic tinge, purpura, bruising, brown discolouration of nails, evidence of excoriation, peripheral oedema, hypertension,

pericardial rub, evidence of pleural effusions, proximal myopathy, evidence of preparation for renal replacement therapy (e.g. arteriovenous fistula, Tenckhoff catheter). **(1 mark for each, max 3 marks)**

3.  Blood and dialysis fluid flow either side of a semipermeable membrane, molecules diffuse down their concentration gradients, plasma biochemistry changes to become more like the dialysis fluid. **(2)**

4.  Bacterial peritonitis, local infection at catheter site, constipation, failure, sclerosing peritonitis. **(1 mark for each, max 2 marks)**

5.  Six months. **(1)**

6.  Increased risk of skin cancer (SCC) due to long-term immunosuppression. **(1)**

Renal replacement therapy is commonly started in patients with an eGFR < 15 and who are symptomatic. Generally speaking, the three options are haemodialysis, peritoneal dialysis and renal transplant. Haemodialysis involves the formation of an arteriovenous fistula. The patient is then connected to a haemodialysis machine, where their blood and dialysis fluid flow in opposite directions on either side of a semipermeable membrane. Molecules diffuse down their concentration gradients, maintaining normal electrolyte concentrations, a normal extracellular volume and removing nitrogenous waste. Peritoneal dialysis involves the insertion of a Tenckhoff catheter, which allows dialysis fluid to be introduced into the peritoneal cavity. The peritoneal membrane is used as a semipermeable membrane, and molecules again diffuse down their concentration gradients to achieve the same goals. Transplantation is often the treatment of choice, and dialysis may be used until an appropriate donor kidney is found. The transplant may be from a cadaveric donor (a brainstem-dead donor who is still being supported and ventilated), from a non-heart-beating donor, from a living related donor or a live unrelated donor. Patients must be ABO compatible with their donor, and HLA matching increases the chance of graft survival. Lifelong immunosuppressive agents are used following this.

## A³

1.  Secondary hyperparathyroidism. **(1)**

2.  Increase osteoclast activity $\rightarrow$ increased $Ca^{2+}$ and $PO_4^{3-}$ release from bone, increased $Ca^{2+}$ and $PO_4^{3-}$ reabsorption via the kidney,

increased hydroxylation of vitamin D. **(1 mark for each, max 2 marks)**

3. Liver, kidney. **(2)**
4. Renal osteodystrophy. **(1)**
5. Restrict dietary phosphate, phosphate-binders, vitamin D analogues, calcium supplements. **(1 mark for each, max 2 marks)**
6. High. **(1)**
7. High. **(1)**
8. Prolonged secondary hyperparathyroidism causing the parathyroid glands to act autonomously. **(1)**

Renal osteodystrophy is just one of the many complications of chronic kidney disease. It results from reduced hydroxylation of vitamin D at the kidney and reduced excretion of phosphate. Patients present with bone pain, pathological fractures and proximal myopathy. Hyperparathyroidism is also a consequence of this. Reduced hydroxylation of vitamin D leads to hypocalcaemia, because active vitamin D is responsible for increasing calcium reabsorption from the gut and the kidney. In order to increase calcium levels, there is an appropriate rise in PTH – secondary hyperparathyroidism. Prolonged secondary hyperparathyroidism causes the glands to undergo adenomatous or hyperplastic change, and high levels of PTH are released even in the presence of normal or high calcium – tertiary hyperparathyroidism. Other complications include a normocytic anaemia. Erythropoietin is responsible for the production of red blood cells, and is normally produced by the kidneys. In chronic kidney disease, there is reduced production of erythropoietin, resulting in anaemia. This may require treatment with erythropoietin injections.

# A⁴

1. Pre-renal, renal/intrinsic, post-renal. **(1 mark, all 3 required)**
2. Causes:
   - pre-renal – hypovolaemia, sepsis, renal artery stenosis, ACEi, NSAIDs, congestive cardiac failure, cirrhosis **(½ a mark for each, max 1 mark)**
   - renal – acute tubular necrosis, nephrotoxins (including nephrotoxic drugs, contrast-induced nephropathy, myeloma, rhabdomyolysis), vasculitis, glomerulonphritis, haemolytic uraemic syndrome, malignant hypertension, thrombotic

thrombocytopenic purpura, cholesterol emboli, acute
tubulointerstitial nephritis, pre-eclampsia (½ a mark for each,
max 1 mark)

- post-renal – renal calculi, renal tumours, ureteric tumours,
BPH, prostate cancer. (½ a mark for each, max 1 mark)

3. ECG, chest X-ray, renal USS, arterial blood gas, urinalysis.
(1 mark for each, max 2 marks)
4. Pulmonary oedema, hyperkalaemia, haemorrhage. (1 mark for
each, max 2 marks)
5. Refractory pulmonary oedema, persistent/refractory
hyperkalaemia, severe metabolic acidosis, uraemic encephalopathy,
uraemic pericarditis. (1 mark for each, max 2 marks)

Acute kidney injury (AKI)/acute renal failure is a deterioration in renal
function over hours to days. Acute-on-chronic renal failure is a deterioration in the renal function of a patient who has an element of chronic
kidney disease. The causes of acute kidney injury are classified as pre-
renal, renal and post-renal. Pre-renal causes result in hypoperfusion of
the kidney, e.g. hypovolaemia, cardiac failure and sepsis. Renal causes
may be due to acute tubular necrosis (often secondary to many of the
pre-renal causes), vascular disease (e.g. vasculitis), glomerular disease (e.g.
glomerulonephritis) and drugs. Post-renal causes are any cause of urinary
tract obstruction, such as BPH, prostate cancer, renal calculi and tumours
of the urinary tract. A renal ultrasound can rapidly and reliably rule out
an obstruction. Management is by treatment of the underlying cause.

## A5

1. Rhabdomyolysis following prolonged immobility. (1)
2. Acute tubular necrosis. (1)
3. Creatinine kinase. (1)
4. Urinary myoglobin. (1)
5. Muddy brown/granular casts. (1)
6. Metformin (risk of metabolic acidosis), lisinopril (nephrotoxic).
(½ a mark for each drug, ½ a mark for each reason, max
2 marks)
7. Excessive exercise, crush injuries, burns, seizures, neuroleptic
malignant syndrome, drugs (e.g. heroin, Ecstacy, statins),

disorders of muscle (e.g. Duchenne's muscular dystrophy), infections (e.g. influenza, EBV). **(1 mark for each, max 3 marks)**

Rhabdomyolysis is often seen in older patients who live alone, fall and have been found some time later by a friend, relative or carer. Skeletal muscle breakdown results in creatinine kinase (CK), myoglobin and other components of skeletal muscle being released into the bloodstream. High circulating levels of myoglobin are filtered through the glomerulus and precipitate, resulting in obstruction of the tubules. Management is with IV fluid rehydration. Nephrotoxic drugs of patients presenting with acute kidney injury should be stopped on admission so as not damage the kidneys further. ACE inhibitors and metformin were mentioned above as drugs that should be stopped. Other drugs to stop include furosemide and NSAIDs.

# A⁶

1. Tall, tented T waves, widening of the QRS complex, flat P waves, prolonged PR interval. **(1 mark for each, max 3 marks)**
2. 10 mL of 10% calcium gluconate IV over ~5 minutes, IV insulin + dextrose, salbutamol nebulisers. **(1 mark for each, max 3 marks)**
3. ANCA, anti-GBM. **((1 mark for each, max 2 marks)**
4. Steroids. **(1)**
5. Renal biopsy. **(1)**

Hyperkalaemia is a medical emergency. The laboratory often phones through the result if it is grossly abnormal. ECG changes may or may not be seen in a patient with hyperkalaemia. In patients with chronic kidney disease or who are known to have a high-normal $K^+$, ECG changes may not be seen, even with extremely high levels. The ECG changes seen are tall, tented T waves, a prolonged PR interval, flattened P waves and widening of the QRS complexes. A 'sine wave' may progress rapidly to asystole and should be treated immediately. A patient with a $K^+ > 7$ or with ECG changes secondary to hyperkalaemia should be given IV calcium gluconate. This will not lower the $K^+$, but will protect the myocardium. Emergency treatment includes IV insulin, which increases intracellular uptake of $K^+$, and should be given with IV dextrose to avoid hypoglycaemia. Salbutamol nebulisers can also be given to lower the $K^+$ level. If hyperkalaemia remains despite these measures, acute dialysis may be required.

# A⁷

1. Proteinuria (> 3 g/24 hours) + hypoalbuminaemia (< 30 g/L) + oedema **(1 mark, all 3 required)**
2. (a) Minimal change disease; (b) membranous nephropathy. **(1 mark for each, max 2 marks)**
3. Renal biopsy. **(1)**
4. Increased susceptibility to infections, increased risk of thromboembolism, hyperlipidaemia. **(1 mark for each, max 2 marks)**
5. By complication:
   - infections – prompt antibiotic treatment if infections are suspected, pneumococcal vaccination
   - thromboembolism – avoid prolonged bed rest, consider anticoagulation
   - hyperlipidaemia – treat with statin **(1 mark per complication, max 2 marks)**
6. Restrict salt intake, normal protein intake. **(1 mark for each, max 2 marks)**

The commonest cause of nephrotic syndrome in children is minimal change disease, the commonest cause in adulthood is membranous nephropathy and in the elderly the commonest cause is focal segmental glomerulosclerosis. Some form of glomerulonephritis is responsible for the vast majority of cases. Other causes include diabetes, amyloidosis, SLE and drugs. Oedema is the main clinical feature, and hypertension may also be present. The main complications of the nephrotic syndrome are infections, thromboembolic disease and hyperlipidaemia. Patients have increased susceptibility to infections because they lose immunoglobulins in their urine and because they are treated with drugs that cause immunosuppression. Patients should be offered the pneumococcal vaccine. Thromboembolic disease occurs due to loss of certain clotting factors in the urine and increased fibrinogen. Hyperlipidaemia occurs due to the increased synthesis of lipoproteins by the liver as a consequence of hypoalbuminaemia. Management includes dietary salt restriction, diuretics, ACE inhibitors and treating the underlying cause.

# A⁸

1. 256.4 (2(118 + 4.5) + 5.3 + 6.1). **(1)**
2. Low. **(1)**
3. Examine JVP, postural blood pressures, serial weights, examine for peripheral oedema, measure urine output, chest X-ray looking for signs of cardiac failure/pulmonary oedema, analyse U&Es. **(1 mark for each, max 3 marks)**
4. Central pontine myelinolysis. **(1)**
5. Posterior pituitary gland. **(1)**
6. Recruits aquaporin 2 channels to the apical membrane of principal cells of the collecting duct, making it water-permeable. **(1)**
7. Syndrome of inappropriate ADH secretion (SIADH). **(1)**
8. Demeclocycline. **(1)**

Hyponatraemia is common, and is often found as an incidental finding in patients presenting to hospital for other reasons. Symptoms of hyponatraemia will depend on how quickly the level has fallen and how low it is, varying from nausea, malaise and headache to confusion, seizures and coma. There are many causes of hyponatraemia, and the first step to identifying the underlying cause is to work out the patient's volume status, i.e. are they hypovolaemic, euvolaemic or hypervolaemic? Hypervolaemic causes tend to be due to nephrotic syndrome or failure of the heart, liver or kidneys. In patients found to be hypovolaemic, urinary sodium should be measured and will give an indication as to whether the sodium is being lost renally (urinary Na > 20) or extra-renally (urinary Na < 20). Renal losses include Addison's disease, diuretics and the diuretic phase of renal failure. Extra-renal losses include diarrhoea, vomiting, burns and fistulae. In euvolaemic patients, urine osmolality should be requested. If this is low, i.e. < 500 mmol/kg, this may be due to hypothyroidism or water excess, e.g. psychogenic polydipsia. If the urine osmolality is high (> 500 mmol/kg), the likely diagnosis is SIADH. The causes of SIADH are vast, and management often requires treatment of the underlying cause, strict fluid restriction and, occasionally, demeclocycline.

# A⁹

1. *E. coli.* **(1)**
2. Females, pregnancy, diabetes, renal calculi, long-term urinary catheterisation, immunosuppression, post-menopause, sexual intercourse, use of spermicide. **(1 mark for each, max 2 marks)**
3. Nitrites, leucocyte esterase. **(1 mark for each, max 2 marks)**
4. Trimethoprim, nitrofurantoin or amoxicillin **(1)** for 3 days. **(1)**
5. Keep well hydrated, drink plenty of cranberry juice, post-coital voiding, wipe front to back, avoid spermicide. **(1 mark for each, max 3 marks)**

*E. coli* is responsible for the majority of urinary tract infections (UTIs). Simple cystitis is most commonly seen in women of childbearing age and presents with dysuria and urinary frequency. Others at higher risk of UTIs are diabetics, patients with long-term urinary catheters, patients who are immunosuppressed and those with a history of renal calculi. A urine dip often confirms the diagnosis, with urine testing positive for nitrites and leucocyte esterase. In addition, microscopic haematuria may also be seen. With this evidence, antibiotics are often started empirically without sending an MSU, usually trimethoprim or nitrofurantoin. If symptoms recur despite an adequate course of antibiotics, an MSU should be sent. Increasingly, multidrug-resistant forms of *E. coli* are being seen, and if a patient has grown this and is symptomatic, the only option may be admission for IV antibiotics. Various measures, listed above, can be taken to reduce the risk of developing UTIs. Occasionally, prophylactic antibiotics are required to prevent UTIs.

# A¹⁰

1. Assess ABC, full history, full examination, IV access, IV fluids, urine dip, request relevant investigations, start empirical antibiotics, discuss with senior colleagues if necessary. **(1 mark for each, max 4 marks)**
2. FBC, U&Es, CRP, urine MC&S, blood cultures, renal USS. **(½ a mark for each, max 2 marks)**
3. Signs/symptoms: (a) stridor, hoarse voice, obvious swelling of the tongue/throat; (b) tachypnoea, cyanosis, wheeze; (c) tachycardia, hypotension, pale appearance, may feel clammy. **(1 mark for each, max 1 mark per category, max 3 marks total)**
4. Route IM, concentration 1 : 1000, volume 0.5 ml **(1)**

Pyelonephritis is an infection of the renal pelvis and often presents as with fever, rigors, loin pain and vomiting. Most cases are caused by *E. coli*. Investigations should include blood tests looking at renal function for evidence of infection and for a causative organism. Urine should also be cultured to ensure appropriate antibiotics are being used. An ultrasound scan is used to ensure there is no evidence of urinary tract obstruction or other obvious abnormalities. True anaphylaxis to penicillin is relatively rare, but the signs and symptoms can develop rapidly, particularly if given IV. Ten per cent of those who develop anaphylaxis to penicillin also react to cephalosporins and carbapenems. A full ABC assessment should be performed, and treatment is with IM adrenaline, IV chlorpheniramine and IV hydrocortisone, as well as IV fluids and high-flow oxygen. ITU should be informed, as the patient may require intubation and ventilator support.

## A¹¹

1. Definitive diagnosis to guide appropriate management. **(1)**
2. Abnormal coagulation studies, single functioning kidney, systolic BP > 160, diastolic BP > 90, CKD with small kidneys. **(1 mark for each, max 2 marks)**
3. Macroscopic haematuria, haematuria requiring blood transfusion, haematuria requiring angiography or nephrectomy, pain (typically flank pain), haematoma, formation of an arteriovenous aneurysm, infection, death. **(1 mark for each, max 3 marks)**
4. Mesangial proliferation, IgA deposits, C3 deposits. **(1 mark for each, max 1 mark)**
5. Immune thrombocytopenic purpura (ITP), thrombotic thrombocytopenic purpura (TTP), senile purpura, septicaemia (commonly meningococcal), post-transfusion purpura, amyloidosis, steroids, psychogenic purpura, disseminated intravascular coagulation (DIC). **(1 mark for each, max 3 marks)**

A renal biopsy may be used to investigate acute renal failure of unknown cause, investigate glomerulonephritis to obtain a definitive diagnosis, to investigate persistent, heavy proteinuria and to investigate deteriorating renal function in a patient post-transplantation. Bleeding is a major complication, with 10%–20% experiencing macroscopic haematuria and 1%–2% requiring a blood transfusion. In 0.1% of cases, the bleeding ultimately leads to death. For this reason, a normal clotting profile is essential, and patients taking anticoagulants should stop them well in advance of the procedure so as to reduce the risk of bleeding. Following the biopsy, bed rest is advised for a number of hours with a pressure dressing applied. Observations should be monitored closely, looking for signs of hypovolaemia. Patients should avoid heavy lifting and strenuous activity for the following 2 weeks.

# Rheumatology

## A¹

1. Rheumatoid factor, anti-CCP (cyclic citrullinated protein) antibodies. **(1 mark for each, max 1 mark)**
2. Joint swelling, ulnar deviation at the fingers, boutonnière deformity (flexion at PIP, hyperextension at DIP), swan-neck deformity (hyperextension at PIP, flexion at DIP), Z-shaped deformity of the thumb (flexion at 1st MCP joint, hyperextension at interphalangeal joint), wrist subluxation, rupture of extensor tendons, muscle wasting. **(1 mark for each, max 3 marks)**
3. Loss of joint space, soft tissue swelling, juxta-articular osteopenia, bony erosions. **(1 mark for each, max 3 marks)**
4. Scleritis, episcleritis, scleromalacia, lymphadenopathy, pleural effusion, pulmonary fibrosis, pericardial effusion, rheumatoid nodules (elbow, pleura), amyloidosis, vasculitis, anaemia, splenomegaly/Felty's syndrome, peripheral neuropathy, Raynaud's phenomenon, carpal tunnel syndrome. **(½ a mark for each, max 2 marks)**
5. Felty's syndrome. **(1)**

Rheumatoid arthritis is a disabling, chronic inflammatory condition that is characterised by a symmetrical polyarthritis. As well as arthritis, this condition has many non-articular features such as those documented above. Early diagnosis and treatment is important, and all suspected cases should be referred to rheumatology for further assessment and consideration of disease-modifying antirheumatic drugs (DMARDs). In order for the diagnosis to be made, four of the following seven criteria, that can be remembered using the mnemonic RF RISES, are required: +ve rheumatoid factor (R), arthritis of the joints of the fingers and hands (F), rheumatoid nodules (R), involvement of ≥ 3 joints for ≥ 6 weeks (I), morning stiffness > 1 hour (S), erosions/other radiographic changes consistent with rheumatoid arthritis (E) and symmetrical arthritis (S). Complications of rheumatoid arthritis include septic arthritis, ruptured tendons, spinal cord compression and side effects of medication used to treat the condition.

# A²

1. Osteoarthritis, psoriatic arthritis, reactive arthritis, Reiter's syndrome, SLE, viral infections (e.g. parvovirus B19), enteropathic arthropathy, endocarditis, systemic conditions (e.g. haemochromatosis, sickle-cell anaemia, malignancy). **(1 mark for each, max 3 marks)**
2. Cyclooxygenase (COX) inhibition → reduces prostaglandin synthesis → reduces inflammation. **(2 marks for adequate explanation)**
3. Orally/intramuscular, once weekly. **(1 mark for route, 1 mark for frequency)**
4. Folic acid **(1)**
5. Rheumatology specialist nurse, physiotherapist, occupational therapist, orthopaedic surgeon. **(1 mark for each, max 2 marks)**

Evidence has shown that early treatment of rheumatoid arthritis, particularly with DMARDs, improves symptoms and long-term outcomes. Methotrexate is commonly used in patients with this condition, but is avoided in pregnancy and in those with liver disease due to its hepatotoxicity. Sulfasalazine, a 5-ASA, is an alternative first-line agent. Biological agents, such as anti-TNFα drugs, are being increasingly used. Steroids are useful for short-term treatment and for 'flares' of the disease, but are not recommended for long-term use. NSAIDs, such as naproxen or ibuprofen, are often required daily to control symptoms, but should be used in caution with those with symptoms of dyspepsia. In those with a history of peptic ulcer disease, a proton pump inhibitor (PPI) should be used in combination for gastric protection. Physiotherapy and surgery also play key roles.

# A³

1. Gout. **(1)**
2. Starting bendroflumethiazide. **(1)**
3. Surgery, starvation/dehydration, alcohol, trauma, infection, aspirin, foods rich in purine. **(1 mark for each, max 3 marks)**
4. Answers: (a) acute – colchicine, steroids, NSAIDS; (b) long-term – allopurinol, sulfinpyrazone, febuxostat. **(1 mark for one acute drug, 1 mark for one long-term drug)**
5. Normal joint space, soft tissue swelling (acute attack), periarticular erosions (later change). **(1 mark for each, max 2 marks)**

6. Negatively birefringent needle shaped crystals **(1)**

Gout is associated with a raised plasma urate, and the symptoms experienced are due to urate crystals being deposited in and around joints. Acute gout causes severe pain, swelling and erythema, is usually monoarticular and classically affects the big toe of middle-aged males. Common triggers of acute gout are trauma, surgery and starting diuretics. Joint radiographs show soft tissue swelling and erosion of periarticular bone but a normal joint space. Acute gout tends to settle on its own after 7 days or so, but NSAIDs are commonly given to relieve inflammation and pain. Colchicine is an alternative. Allopurinol reduces serum urate and is used to prevent acute attacks. Introducing allopurinol itself, however, can precipitate an attack. It is therefore advised to wait for 3 weeks after an attack before starting it and to use colchicine or an NSAID as cover initially. Chronic tophaceous gout is seen in individuals with high levels of urate over long periods of time. In this condition, urate forms tophi (smooth white deposits) which are seen in the pinna, tendons and joints.

## A⁴

1. Chondrocalcinosis. **(1)**
2. Pseudogout. **(1)**
3. Hips, wrist **(1 mark for each, max 2 marks)**
4. Hypothyroidism, hyperparathyroidism, haemochromatosis, Wilson's disease, OA, increasing age. **(1 mark for each, max 2 marks)**
5. Polarised light microscopy of synovial fluid. **(1)**
6. Weakly positively birefringent rhomboid-shaped crystals. **(1)**
7. Septic arthritis, gout, trauma, reactive arthritis. **(1 mark for each, max 2 marks)**

Pseudogout is caused by the deposition of calcium pyrophosphate in cartilage. It presents in a similar way to gout, although affects different joints, commonly the knee or wrist, and is commoner in elderly women. Radiographs may reveal calcium deposition, but the diagnosis is ultimately made by identifying weakly positive birefringent crystals in synovial fluid. Pseudogout often resolves spontaneously, but if it fails to settle, NSAIDs and other simple analgesics are used. Younger people presenting with this condition often have risk factors for the condition, such as Wilson's disease or hyperparathyroidism.

# A⁵

1. Antalgic gait, varus deformity, joint swelling/effusion, joint tenderness, crepitus, fixed flexion deformity, muscle wasting, reduced range of movement, pain on movement at the joint. **(1 mark for each, max 4 marks)**

2. Loss of joint space, osteophytes, subchondral sclerosis, subchondral cysts. **(½ a mark for each, max 2 marks)**

3. Conservative (weight loss, exercise), physiotherapy, simple analgesia, opioid analgesia, intra-articular injections, surgical (joint replacement). **(1 mark for each, max 4 marks)**

Osteoarthritis often presents with pain, stiffness, crepitus and joint swelling in the older populations. Commonly affected joints are the hips, knees and joints of the hands. Radiographs classically show narrowing of the joint space, osteophyte formation, subchondral sclerosis and subchondral cysts. Conservative management should be trialled first. This includes encouraging weight loss, physiotherapy and the use of walking aids/supportive footwear, etc. Medical management may involve oral or topical analgesia and intra-articular injections. In severe osteoarthritis, operations are performed to replace the affected joint.

# A⁶

1. ANA, anti-dsDNA, anti-Sm, antiphospholipid antibodies (anti-cardiolipin and lupus anticoagulants), rheumatoid factor. **(1 mark for each, max 2 marks)**

2. Malar rash, discoid rash, photosensitive rash, vasculitic rash. **(1 mark for each, max 2 marks)**

3. Antiphospholipid syndrome. **(1)**

4. Coagulation defects, livedo reticularis, thrombocytopenia. **(1 mark for each, max 3 marks)**

5. Aspirin, warfarin, clopidogrel, heparin. **(1 mark for each, max 2 marks)**

Systemic lupus erythematosis is an autoimmune, multisystemic condition that commonly takes a relapsing-remitting course. The majority of patients have a positive ANA titre, and many test positive for anti-dsDNA antibodies which are almost entirely specific to SLE. The most commonly affected sites are the joints and skin. NSAIDs or hydroxychloroquine are commonly used to control symptoms affecting these sites, and many also require long-term low-dose steroids. Intensive immuno-suppression is required for lupus nephritis, and many patients eventually require some form of renal replacement therapy. Antiphospholipid syndrome (APLS) is seen in 20%–30% of those with SLE. The features seen can be remembered by the mnemonic CLOT: Coagulation defects, Livedo reticularis, Obstetric problems (recurrent miscarriage) and Thrombocytopenia. Patients with APLS test positive for anticardiolipin antibodies and lupus anticoagulants. If patients suffer recurrent thrombo-ses, they usually receive warfarin with a target INR range of 2–3.

## A⁷

1. Heliotrope. **(1)**
2. Gottron's papules. **(1)**
3. Anti-Jo-1, anti-Mi-2, rheumatoid factor, ANA. **(1 mark for each, max 2 marks)**
4. Peripheral digital ischaemia caused by vasospasm which is precipitated by cold or emotion. **(1)**
5. Raynaud's disease, SLE, RA, dermatomyositis/polymyositis, Ehlers–Danlos syndrome, β-blockers, polycythaemia rubra vera, occupational causes (e.g. using vibrating tools), MGUS, hypothyroidism, atherosclerosis, thoracic outlet obstruction, Buerger's disease, cold agglutinin disease. **(1 mark for each, max 3 marks)**
6. Calcinosis, oesophageal dysmotility, sclerodactly, telangiectasia **(½ a mark for each, max 2 marks)**

Polymyositis and dermatomyositis both cause progressive proximal muscle weakness, but dermatomyositis also causes skin signs, such as heliotrope (a purple rash on the eyelids) and Gottron's papules (red papules over the knuckles, elbows and knees). Anti-Jo-1 and anti-Mi-2 antibodies are positive in patients with these conditions. Both are asso-ciated with an increased risk of malignancy, and screening should be performed regularly. Management is usually with steroids, but immuno-suppressive agents and cytotoxic drugs may be required if the response to steroids is not adequate. Systemic sclerosis may be limited, i.e. the CREST syndrome, or diffuse, in which there is disease involving the lungs, kidneys and heart. Immunosuppressive agents again form the mainstay of treatment.

# A⁸

1. Psoriatic arthritis, reactive arthritis, enteropathic arthritis, Reiter's syndrome. **(1 mark for each, max 2 marks)**
2. HLA-B27. **(1)**
3. Calcification of intervertebral ligaments, fusion of spinal facet joints and formation of bridging syndesmophytes – the so-called bamboo spine. **(1 mark for each, max 2 marks)**
4. NSAIDs, intra-articular injections, anti-TNFα drugs (e.g. etanercept, infliximab, adalimumab). **(1 mark for each, max 2 marks)**
5. Anterior uveitis/iritis. **(1)**
6. Early diastolic murmur (aortic regurgitation), fine inspiratory crepitations, commonly at apices (pulmonary fibrosis). **(1 mark for each, max 2 marks)**

Ankylosing spondylitis is typically seen in young adult males and presents insidiously with low back pain and morning stiffness, and the majority of patients test positive for HLA-B27. Many cases progress to cause thoracic kyphosis and hyperextension of the neck, giving the classical 'question mark' posture. NSAIDs are commonly used for pain, exercise programmes are available to ensure posture and mobility are maintained and prolonged rest is not advised. Other management options include intra-articular injections and joint replacement surgery in severe cases. There are numerous extra-articular associations also, including aortic regurgitation, pulmonary fibrosis, anterior uveitis and amyloidosis.

# A⁹

1. Flexural psoriasis, guttate psoriasis, erythrodermic psoriasis, pustular psoriasis. **(1 mark for each, max 2 marks)**
2. Extensor surfaces of arms, extensor surfaces of legs, ears, scalp, lower back. **(½ a mark for each, max 1 mark)**
3. Arthritis mutilans. **(1)**
4. *Chlamydia, Ureaplasma, Campylobacter, Salmonella, Shigella, Yersinia.* **(1 mark for each, max 3 marks)**
5. Conjunctivitis, urethritis, arthritis. **(1 mark for each, max 3 marks)**

Psoriatic arthritis affects approximately 10% of those with psoriasis, and can present in a number of forms. Most commonly, psoriatic arthritis affects the distal interphalangeal joints. Dactylitis, inflammation of an entire digit, is a feature of this, and gives rise to the 'sausage finger' seen in these patients. Other forms include a symmetrical arthritis that presents in a similar fashion to rheumatoid arthritis, and arthritis mutilans. In this severe form of the condition, the appearances are often more severe than the symptoms experienced by the patient. Reactive arthritis is a sterile arthritis that is typically seen soon after urethritis or a diarrhoeal infection. The commonest organisms that cause this have been listed above. Reiter's syndrome is a form of reactive arthritis. The features of this can be rememberd by the rhyme 'Can't see (conjunctivitis), can't pee (urethritis) and can't climb up a tree (arthritis)'.

## A¹⁰

1. ANCA +ve (microscopic polyangiitis, Churg-Strauss syndrome), ANCA –ve (Henoch–Schönlein purpura, cryoglobulinaemia, Goodpasture's disease). **(1 mark for 1 correct answer from each category, max 2 marks)**

2. Large (temporal arteritis, Takayasu's arteritis), medium (polyarteritis nodosa, Kawasaki's disease). **(1 mark for 1 correct answer from each category, max 2 marks)**

3. Infective endocarditis, rheumatoid arthritis, Behçet's, SLE, inflammatory bowel disease, scleroderma, hepatitis B and C, polymyositis, dermatomyositis. **(1 mark for each, max 2 marks)**

4. HIV/AIDS, rheumatoid arthritis, diabetes, sarcoidosis, polyarteritis nodosa, leprosy, carcinomatosis. **(1 mark for each, max 4 marks)**

Inflammation of the blood vessel walls is known as vasculitis. Vasculitis is classified according to the size of the vessel involved. Temporal arteritis is a form of large-vessel vasculitis that has already been discussed. Takayasu's arteritis causes vasculitis of the aortic arch and other major arteries, and is uncommon in the UK. Medium-vessel vasculitides include polyarteritis nodosa (PAN), which is again rare in the UK and may be associated with hepatitis B. Unusually for vasculitis, PAN affects males more frequently than females. Kawasaki's disease is another form of medium-vessel vasculitis. This is most commonly seen in children under the age of 5, and if not detected early it may cause coronary artery aneurysms. Small-vessel vasculitis can be subcategorised as those that are ANCA +ve and those that are ANCA –ve. Wegener's, Churg-Strauss and microscopic polyangiitis are all ANCA +ve. Henoch–Schönlein purpura, cryoglobulinaemia and Goodpasture's disease are all ANCA –ve. Steroids are the mainstay of treatment for large-vessel vasculitis, and are often used in conjunction with immunosuppressive agents to treat medium- and small-vessel vasculitis. Many systemic illnesses can cause vasculitis, and these are listed above.

# Endocrinology

## A¹

1. Hypersecretion of growth hormone by a tumour in the anterior pituitary gland in adulthood. **(1)**
2. Thick spade-like hands, frontal bossing, macroglossia, bitemporal hemianopia, headache, sweats, wide-spaced teeth, prognathism, voice changes, sleep disturbance due to obstructive sleep apnoea, carpal tunnel syndrome, increased blood pressure. **(½ a mark for each, max 3 marks)**
3. Bitemporal hemianopia due to pituitary tumour pressing on optic chiasm. **(1)**
4. Serum insulin-like growth factor 1 (IGF-1). **(1)**
5. Rapid increase in blood glucose should suppress growth hormone secretion. This will not occur in a patient with acromegaly. **(1)**
6. Diabetes mellitus because growth hormone is an anti-insulin and this leads to a state of insulin resistance and eventually diabetes. **(1)**
7. Cardiovascular disease. **(1)**
8. Transsphenoidal resection of pituitary tumour. **(1)**

Over 95% of cases of acromegaly are due to a pituitary tumour; other causes are from ectopic production from other tumours, particularly carcinoid. A useful aid in examining patients is to ask for old photos of themselves as well as to look for the signs and symptoms as mentioned in the answers section. Serum IGF-1 is the blood test performed and is raised in acromegaly. It is produced in the liver secondary to high levels of growth hormone. Random assays of growth hormone are not used, as it has a short half-life and is secreted in a pulsatile manner. An OGTT with the lack of suppression of growth hormone secretion is diagnostic. MRI is the choice of imaging of the pituitary. Cardiovascular disease is the major cause of death secondary to increase in heart muscle size, raised blood pressure and insulin resistance.

# A²

1. Amiodarone, radiotherapy. (½ **a mark for each, max 1 mark**)
2. Dry/thinning hair, bradycardia, dry skin, loss of lateral third of eyebrows, ataxia, mental slowness, goitre, carpal tunnel syndrome, oedema, peaches-and-cream complexion, slow relaxing reflexes, peripheral neuropathy. (½ **a mark for each, max 2 marks**)
3. Autoimmune, iodine deficiency, cancer, infection, hypopituitarism. (**1 mark for each, max 2 marks**)
4. Macrocytic anaemia. (**1**)
5. TSH high, $T_4$ low. (**1**)
6. Levothyroxine. (**1**)
7. Vitiligo. (**1**)
8. Foramen caecum. (**1**)

Hypothyroidism is a relatively common condition. It has many causes, but most commonly it is autoimmune in nature, leading to atrophy and eventually fibrosis by autoantibodies. It is associated with other autoimmune conditions, such as vitiligo or pernicious anaemia. Iatrogenic causes such as antithyroid drugs like amiodarone or lithium can also be the cause. Other causes are congenital agenesis, post-partum thyroiditis, infective (usually after a period of hyperthyroidism), radioactive iodine therapy or thyroidectomy. Secondary hypothyroidism can be caused by hypopituitarism. A large list of symptoms and signs are characteristic. Another possible treatment in this lady would be to do a trial of stopping amiodarone and monitoring; however, specialist advice would be needed from a cardiologist.

# A³

1. Autoimmune disease caused by TSH receptor antibodies. (**1**)
2. Tachycardia, fast irregular heartbeat (AF), warm peripheries, goitre, ophthalmoplegia, pretibial myxoedma, thyroid acropatchy, palmar erythema, thinning of the hair, brisk reflexes, lid lag, exophthalmos, high-output cardiac failure signs. (**1 mark for each, max 3 marks**)
3. Low TSH, high $T_4$. (**1**)
4. β-blocker. (**1**)
5. Propythiouracil, carbimazole. (**1 mark for each, max 2 marks**)

6. Pretibial myxoedema, eye disease (ophthalmoplegia/ exophthalmos), thyroid acropatchy. **(1 mark for each, max 2 marks)**

Hyperthyroidism, particularly Graves' disease, is much commoner in females. The TSH receptor antibodies cause a stimulatory effect on the thyroid, increasing the levels of circulatory thyroxine and causing a diffuse enlargement of the thyroid gland, which is clinically apparent as a goitre. It is associated with other autoimmune disease such as Addison's and diabetes mellitus. Specific to Graves' are the three signs mentioned above. The antibodies cause oedema of the eye muscle, giving the signs of ophthalmoplegia, which is most noticeable when a patient is asked to look up. Smoking worsens thyroid eye disease, so patients should be advised to quit.

# A⁴

1. Diabetes insipidus. **(1)**
2. Posterior pituitary. **(1)**
3. Urine osmolality – low; plasma osmolality – high. **(1 mark for each)**
4. Nephrogenic – in the kidney, there is resistence/lack of response to ADH; cranial – there is lack of/insufficient production of ADH. **(1 mark for each)**
5. Patient is starved of any fluid intake. **(1)** The normal response of the body would be to concentrate urine and decrease urine output; however, in diabetes insipidus, there is continued production of large volumes of urine with low osmolality. **(1)**
6. Desmopressin. **(1)**
7. Sheehan's syndrome (pituitary infarction). **(1)**

Diabetes insipidus (DI) has a very similar presentation to diabetes mellitus. It is divided into cranial and nephrogenic, each with a large list of causes. Large volumes of dilute urine after deprivation of water is diagnostic, and the two types can be distinguished with administration of desmopressin during the test. After desmopressin is given, if large volumes continue to be produced, nephrogenic DI must be suspected. If urine volume drops and becomes more concentrated, then cranial DI is suspected. The main treatment in both cases is to look for the underlying cause.

# A⁵

1. Blood glucose testing. **(1)**
2. IM glucagons, IV glucose. **(1 mark for each)**
3. Administering insulin (overmedicating). **(1)**
4. Confusion, drowsiness, seizures, hemiparesis. **(1 mark for each, max 2 marks)**
5. A lack of awareness of hypoglycaemia. **(1)**
6. Regular finger-prick monitoring; never miss a meal; keep 'emergency supply' of glucose in pocket, e.g. energy tablets; adjust insulin appropriately in response to change in diet, activity, illness. **(1 mark for each, max 2 marks)**
7. Liver failure, Addison's, insulin-secreting tumours, alcohol binging, pituitary insufficiency. **(1 mark for each, max 1 mark)**

Hypoglycaemia is the commonest diabetic emergency. Patients usually go through an initial stage, with autonomic symptoms such as sweating, palpitations and tremor, but with further decline in blood glucose, neuroglycopenia sets in, as in the case above. With repeated exposure to hypoglycaemic states, the body can 'lose awareness', and the initial autonomic symptoms do not occur. Treatment is usually with IV glucose in the situations described in the question; however, if a patient is able to take things orally, then the oral route is the preferred route with high-glucose-containing gels or drinks.

# A⁶

1. Type 2 diabetes mellitus. **(1)**
2. Any three of the following:
   - patient fasts overnight prior to test
   - a drink containing 75 g of glucose in 300 ml of water is given
   - blood glucose is measured prior to the drink and then at 120 minutes (interval samples can also be taken)
   - diabetes is diagnosed if blood glucose at 120 minutes is > 11.1 mmol/L
   - diabetes can also be diagnosed if the fasting blood glucose sample is > 7 mmol/L
   - patient is adviced not to drink coffee or smoke in fasting period. **(3)**

3. Macrovascular: cerebrovascular disease/stroke, myocardial infarction/ischaemic heart disease, peripheral vascular disease. (½ a mark for each, max. 1 mark)

   Microvascular: nephropathy, neuropathy, retinopathy. (½ a mark for each, max 1 mark)

4. Biguanides (metformin), thiazolidinediones (rosiglitazone), sulphonylureas (tolbutamide), meglitinides (repaglinide), alpha-glucosidase inhibitors, insulin. (1 mark for each, max 3 marks)

5. Lifestyle advice – lose weight, eat healthily, stop smoking. (1)

This example is of the subacute presentation of type 2 diabetes. Patients may not always have the full-blown triad of weight loss, polydipsia and polyuria. It can also mean that patients can present with advanced complications of the disease, such as blurred vision. The key to managing diabetes is with patient education and advice on the seriousness of the condition, as cardiovascular disease is the largest cause of death in diabetic patients. The goal of treatment is to maintain good glycaemic control, as this reduces complications.

# A7

1. Urine dipstick – presence of ketonuria. (1)
2. FBC (may indicate infection), U&E (electrolyte abnormality and renal failure). (1 mark for each, max 2 marks)
3. Metabolic acidosis with respiratory compensation. (1)
4. Fluid replacement (aggressively), insulin sliding scale, potassium replacement (1 mark for each, max 3 marks)
5. Insulin deficiency produces glucose production in the liver; lipolysis also occurs; fatty acids are broken done to form ketone bodies which produce a metabolic acidosis. (1 mark for each)

Diabetic ketoacidosis may be the first presentation of diabetes in a patient. The severe metabolic acidosis causes the body to compensate with hyperventilation (Kussmaul's respiration), and the acidosis also causes the patient to vomit, which causes further fluid loss and electrolyte disturbance. This gives the clinical picture as described in the question. The patient also has polyuria secondary to glucose-induced osmotic diuresis and may complain of abdominal pain. The first and most vital step in management is fluid replacement, as it is the fluid depletion that is the most immediate threat to life. Electrolytes must be monitored, in particular potassium, as insulin causes a peripheral uptake into the tissues.

## A⁸

1. Addison's disease, autoimmune. **(1 mark for each)**
2. U&E, Synacthen test. **(1 mark for each)**
3. Low sodium, high potassium. **(1 mark for each)**
4. Mineralocorticoids. **(1)**
5. Carry a steroid card; medic alert bracelet; know how to change dose of medication for intercurrent illness; carry an emergency ampoule of hydrocortisone for when oral route is not advisable. **(1 mark for each, max 3 marks)**

Addison's disease is rare. The commonest cause worldwide is adrenal TB infection; in the UK, the commonest cause is autoimmune. It can present sometimes in Addison's crises, whereby the patient can be hypotensive, hyperkalaemic, hypoglycaemic and hyponatraemic. This is why patients should carry steroid cards and medic alert bracelets explaining details of their steroid dependency in case of being found collapsed.

## A⁹

1. Prolactinoma. **(1)**
2. Galactorrhoea, decreased libido, subfertility, headache, visual field defect. **(1 mark for each, max 3 marks)**
3. MRI head. **(1)**
4. Prolactinoma may grow and press upon the optic chiasm **(1)** causing a bitemporal hemianopia. **(1)**
5. Cabergoline/bromocriptine, dopamine agonist. **(1 mark for each)**
6. Radiotherapy. **(1)**

Hyperprolactinaemia has many causes, such as prolactinoma, stalk compression from other pituitary tumours, hypothyroidism, polycystic ovarian syndrome and iatrogenic secondary to medication such as haloperidol. Transsphenoidal resection surgery is a good option for microadenomas. Radiotherapy has the adverse effect of causing hypopituitarism. Dopamine agonism decreases prolactin secretion. Bromocriptine is the drug of choice if planning for a pregnancy.

# A¹⁰

1. Polydipsia, polyuria, signs of dehydration, weakness, depression, constipation, signs of renal stones, signs of pancreatitis, bone pain. **(1 mark for each, max 3 marks)**
2. Parathyroid hormone level. **(1)**
3. Low. **(1)**
4. DEXA scan, isotope scan, ultrasound, abdominal X-ray, CT/MRI neck. **(1 mark for each, max 2 marks)**
5. Hypoparathryroidism, laryngeal nerve palsy. **(1 mark for each)**
6. Vitamin D is needed to absorb calcium in the gut. **(1)**

The commonest cause of hyperparathyroidism is adenoma. Patients present with very vague symptoms, but markedly elevated levels of calcium, polydipsia and polyuria can be present, so it is important to rule out diabetes with a simple urine dipstick. After finding an elevated calcium level without any obvious cause, the next most appropriate investigation is to measure the parathyroid hormone level. If this is normal, malignancy must be excluded.

# A¹¹

1. 'Glove and stocking' distribution. **(1)**
2. Vibration sense. **(1)**
3. Charcot's joint/neuropathic arthropathy/joint deformity; painless ulcer; high arched foot with clawing of the toes; diminished reflexes. **(1 mark for each, max 3 marks)**
4. Autonomic neuropathy; diabetic amyotrophy; mononeuropathy/ mononeuritis multiplex; acute painful neuropathy. **(1 mark for each, max 2 marks)**
5. Good glycaemic control. **(1)**
6. Eyes – ophthalmological assessment; kidneys – renal investigation. **(1 mark for each)**
7. Autonomic gastroparesis. **(1)**

This case demonstrates one of the microvascular complications of diabetes – neuropathy. Patients can develop joint deformity due to repeated minor injury to the feet, and ulcers can develop because of a lack of awareness of any injury. Patients rely on visual proprioception to move around, so in the dark, patients are at risk of falling. It is important to investigate other microvascular complications, as the presence of one nearly invariably means presence of the other two.

# Haematology

## A¹

1. Night sweats, weight loss, itching, fever, tiredness, alcohol-induced pain at node sites. **(1 mark for each, max 3 marks)**
2. Enlargement of nodes at other site, splenomegaly; hepatomegaly. **(1 mark for each)**
3. Reed-Sternberg cell. **(1)**
4. CXR, CT chest /abdomen/pelvis, bone marrow biopsy. **(1 mark for each, max 2 marks)**
5. Ann Arbor. **(1)**
6. Superior vena cava obstruction. **(1)**

The cause for the enlarged lymph node in Daniel is due to malignant proliferation of lymphocytes which have accumulated there. Patients with lymphoma may be asymptomatic or complain of 'B' symptoms, such as nights sweats, weight loss and fever. These 'B' symptoms suggest more advanced disease. The Reed-Sternberg cell is pathognomonic of Hodgkin's lymphoma. Imaging and marrow biopsy is required to fully stage the disease so treatment can be planned appropriately. Superior vena cava obstruction in this patient would be caused by mediastinal lymph node enlargement.

## A²

1. Microcytic anaemia. **(2)**
2. Tachypnoea, pale conjunctiva, tachycardia, ejection systolic murmur. **(1 mark for each, max 3 marks)**
3. Poor diet, malabsorption, e.g. coeliacs, hookworm infection, chronic bleeding from any other source. **(1)**
4. Angular cheilosis, koilionychia; atrophic glossitis. **(1 mark for each)**
5. Black stools, constipation, diarrhoea, nausea. **(1 mark for each, max 2 marks)**

Microcytic anaemia is low haemoglobin and low mean cell volume. Causes include thalassaemia, sideroblastic anaemia and lead poisoning, but iron deficiency is by far the commonest cause. Iron-deficiency anaemia is most commonly caused by blood loss. Iron studies can be done to confirm diagnosis. They would show a low serum ferritin and iron with a raised total iron-binding capacity. Signs of severe anaemia are those associated with a hyperdynamic circulation. Signs more specific to iron-deficiency anaemia are mentioned above. Koilonychia is seen as spooning of the nails, angular cheilosis is splitting and cracking of the skin at the corner of the mouth, usually bilaterally, and atrophic glossitis appears as a smoothness to the tongue surface as there is loss of the papillae.

## A³

1. Hydroxyurea (hydroxycarbamide), penicillin, folic acid. (**1 mark for each, max 2 marks**)
2. Exposure to cold, dehydration, hypoxia, acidosis. (**1 mark for each, max 2 marks**)
3. Oxygen, analgesia, intravenous fluids, empirical antibiotics. (**1 mark for each, max 3 marks**)
4. Autosomal recessive. (**1**)
5. 100%. (**1**)
6. High levels of foetal haemoglobin (Hb F) which mask the effect of the disease until levels of Hb F begin to fall at 6 months old. (**1**)

Sickle-cell disease is an autosomal recessive disease most commonly found in Africans. It is called sickle-cell disease when it is in its homozygous state (Hb SS) and is called sickle-cell trait in the heterozygous state (Hb AS). Different types of crises can present, most serious of which is acute chest syndrome, which is associated with a relatively high mortality rate. After deoxygenation, the red blood cells become stiff and sickle-shaped, which can lead to vaso-occlusion of the small blood vessels causing the crises. With long-standing disease, patients can go through 'autosplenectomy' because of repeated infarcts in the spleen. This leaves them vulnerable to encapsulated bacteria, so they are given prophylactic penicillin. Sickle-cell disease is protective against malaria.

## A⁴

1. Malignant clonal proliferation of β-lymphocytic plasma cells. (**1**)
2. IgG. (**1**)

3.  Recurrent infections, bruising easily, tiredness, polydipsia, abdominal pain, bone pain, confusion. **(1 mark for each, max 2 marks)**

4.  FBC, blood film, U&E, serum electrophoresis, urine electrophoresis, serum calcium, serum immunoglobulins, bone marrow sampling. **(1 mark for each, max 3 marks)**

5.  Possible bone marrow infiltration; immunoparesis secondary to overexpression of one immunoglobulin and underexpression of any other immunoglobulins. **(1 mark for each)**

6.  Hypercalcaemia, spinal cord compression, hyperviscosity, acute renal failure. **(½ a mark for each, max 2 marks)**

Myeloma is a monoclonal expansion of the B-lymphocytic plasma cells, which overexpress one type of immunoglobulin. In the majority of cases, it is IgG which is overexpressed. This overexpression causes diminished production of any other immunoglobulin, giving an immunoparesis and hence susceptibility to bacterial infections. The malignant cells also produce osteoclast-activating factors which lead to crush fractures, such as the patient presented with. Diagnosis is found when a monoclonal band is found of electrophoresis in combination with evidence of increased plasma cells in the bone marrow and evidence of end organ damage, such as renal failure or bone lesions. In some cases, it can present as one of the four acute complications mentioned.

# A5

1.  Malaria, myelofibrosis, lymphoma, liver cirrhosis with portal hypertension, haemolytic anaemia, mononucleosis, amyloidosis. **(1 mark for each, max 3 marks)**

2.  High. **(1)**

3.  Chronic leukaemia will show white cells which are mature and the full spectrum of lineage; acute leukaemia shows only white cells in the blast stage (immature). **(2)**

4.  Philadelphia chromosome. **(1)**

5.  Imatinib, tyrosine kinase inhibitor, oral route. **(1 mark for each)**

6.  Trial of different tyrosine kinase inhibitor, bone marrow transplant. **(1 mark for each)**

CML is a disease that usually affects the middle-aged to elderly population. It can present with shortness of breath, tiredness, fullness in the abdomen, weight loss and fever. The full blood count usually shows a lymphocytosis. The blood film will show a spectrum of maturity. A bone marrow sample at this stage is required, and on gentetic testing in the vast majority of cases will show the characteristic BCR-ABL translocation between chromosomes 9 and 22, the Philadelphia chromosome. Treatment is now outpatient-based due to the breakthrough of the tyrosine kinase inhibitor imatinib (Glivec) in the past decade. Other tyrosine kinase inhibitors are now available, which can be trialled after initial poor response to imatinib, or a bone marrow transplant can be performed.

## A⁶

1. Leucopenia/neutropenia, thrombocytopenia, anaemia. **(1 mark for each, max 3 marks)**
2. Marrow infiltration. **(1)**
3. Blood film (looking for the presence of immature blast cells). **(1)**
4. Acute **(1)** myeloid leukaemia. **(1)**
5. Blood transfusions to help with symptoms of anaemia; platelet transfusions to prevent haemorrhage; prophylactic and treatment with antibiotics/antivirals/antifungals; counselling about the diagnosis and treatment implications. **(1 mark for each, max 3 marks)**

With acute leukaemia, patients usually present with the signs of bone marrow failure, symptoms of anaemia, bleeding (due to thrombocytopenia) and symptoms of infection (because of leucopenia). Patients can become rapidly unwell in a matter of days. Acute leukaemia is associated with exposure to radiation and also chemical exposure such as benzene. A blood film will always show blast cells and lineage can be confirmed on immunophenotyping. The mainstay of treatment of acute leukaemia is with chemotherapy and stem cell transplantation. However, patients will require long hospital stays during the active phases of their treatment, where there is a need for supportive care measures as mentioned above.

## A⁷

1. 7 g/dL. **(1)**
2. Tachycardia, tachypnoea, flow murmur, pallor. **(1 mark for each, max 2 marks)**
3. Acute haemolytic reaction, bacterial contamination. **(1 mark for each)**

4. Stop the transfusion. **(1)**
5. Disseminated intravascular coagulation. **(1)**
6. Early: acute haemolytic reaction, bacterial contamination, allergic reaction, anaphalaxis, transfusion-related acute lung injury, fluid overload, non-haemolytic febrile transfusion reaction. **(1)**

   Late: iron overload, graft versus host disease, post-transfusion purpura, infection. **(1)**
7. Transfusion of the entire patient's blood volume/10 units of blood **(1)** within 24 hours. **(1)**

Blood transfusion reactions are rare but can be fatal. The usual cause is human error: giving the wrong blood product to the wrong patient. In these cases, usually an acute haemolytic transfusion reaction can occur like the one described above; rapid onset with fever and hypotension. A complicating factor is the possibility of disseminated intravascular coagulation. The initial step is to stop the transfusion. The blood product should be sent back to the lab and a repeat sample should be cross-matched to confirm it was the correct blood product given. Massive blood transfusion has added complications, such as hypocalcaemia, hypothermia, hyperkalaemia and a dilutional effect on the other components of blood, causing a thrombocytopenia.

# A⁸

1. Megaloblastic **(1)**: vitamin $B_{12}$ deficiency, folate deficiency, cytotoxic drugs. **(2)**

   Non-megaloblastic **(1)**: alcohol, liver disease, hypothyroidism, pregnancy, reticulocytosis. **(2)**
2. Blood film. **(1)**
3. Pernicious anaemia. **(1)**
4. Parietal cell antibody serology, intrinsic factor antibody serology, Schilling test. **(1 mark for each, max 1 mark)**
5. Intramuscular hydroxycobalamin. **(1)**

Macrocytic anaemia is diagnosed with finding a high MCV with low haemoglobin on full blood count. It has many causes, such as the ones mentioned above, and can be divided into megaloblastic and non-megaloblastic. A megaloblast is a large nuclear red blood cell. A simple blood film will reveal if any megaloblasts are present. Pernicious anaemia is the commonest cause for megaloblastic macrocytic anaemia. It is an autoimmune disease, causing a lack of intrinsic factor due to autoimmune destruction of gastric parietal cells. Parietal cell antibodies are found in 90% of pernicious anaemia cases. Folate deficiency is another common cause for megaloblastic anaemia. There are four causes of deficiency: poor diet, e.g in vegans; increased demand occurring, e.g. in pregnancy; malabsorption, notably in coeliac disease; anti-folate drugs, e.g. methotrexate.

# A⁹

1. Hypochromic **(1)** microcytic **(1)** anaemia. **(1)**
2. Hepatosplenomegaly, frontal bossing, jaw enlargement, dental malocclusion, flow murmur, generalised pallor, conjunctival pallor, tachycardia. **(1 mark for each, max 2 marks)**
3. Cooley's anaemia. **(1)**
4. Blood transfusion, iron chelation therapy (e.g. desferrioxamine). **(1 mark for each)**
5. Genetic counselling. **(1)**
6. Due to the large production of foetal haemoglobin in the early part of life, which ceases as the child gets older. **(1)**

The thalassaemias are classified by which one of the haemoglobin chains is affected, with α-thalassaemia the α-chain is affected, and in β-thalassaemia the β-chain is affected. β-thalassaemia is common in Mediterranean countries, with reported incidence of one in eight Cypriot people having the thalassaemia trait (one abnormal globin gene). These patients are usually asymptomatic, but usually have a mild microcytic anaemia on blood testing. β-thalassaemia major has a one-in-four chance of occurring in a child born to parents who both have the thalassaemia trait (this is why genetic counselling should be offered to a couple of Mediterranean origin). They usually present in early childhood, but not immediately at birth due to the prolonged production of foetal haemoglobin. It is important to note that α-thalassaemia major is usually fatal in utero. Serum electrophoresis is needed to confirm diagnosis. Transfusions and iron chelation therapy are the mainstay of treatment for thalassaemia major. Complications of the disease are usually secondary to iron overload; however, these have been reduced since the introduction of iron chelation therapy, with the vast majority of sufferers living well beyond 50 years old.

# A10

1. Compartment syndrome, fasciotomy. **(1 mark for each)**
2. Spontaneous bleeding into joints. **(1)**
3. X-linked recessive. **(1)**
4. VIII. **(1)**
5. INR – normal; APTT – prolonged. **(1 mark for each)**
6. Purified factor VIII, fresh frozen plasma containing factor VIII, desmopressin. **(1 mark for each, max 1 mark)**
7. Acquired haemophilia A. **(1)**

Haemophilia A is the commonest inherited bleeding disorder and is a deficiency of factor VIII. It is inherited in an X-linked recessive pattern, so that the sons of carrier mothers are affected and a clear family history is usually demonstrated. However, rarely, it is acquired with autoantibodies to factor VIII, usually in old age. Complications of the disease usually present in early life, with spontaneous bleeding into joints causing arthropathy. Another acute presentation is with compartment syndrome, as described in the clinical case. Patients are usually monitored by a specific haemophilia service that monitors and administers factor VIII. Advice to these patients should also be given, such as to wear a medic alert bracelet for acute presentations, avoid NSAIDS and intramuscular injections as well as lifestyle advice with regards to avoiding contact sports and other similar activities.

# Gastroenterology

## A¹

1. Inflammatory bowel disease, irritable bowel disease, infective diarrhoea (protozoa/parasites more likely at 3 months), coeliac disease, colorectal carcinoma, medications, chronic pancreatitis, thyrotoxicosis. **(½ a mark for each, max 2 marks)**
2. Basic tests:
   - full blood count may reveal anaemia and a raised white cell count
   - CRP may be raised
   - albumin may be decreased
   - vitamin $B_{12}$ deficiency
   - stool MC&S
   - coeliac screen
   - amylase
   - TFT

   Invasive tests:
   - sigmoidoscopy + rectal biopsy
   - colonoscopy
   - barium enema (may show cobblestoning, strictures and ulcers, but unable to biopsy)
   - capsule endoscopy (for small bowel disease). **(2)**
3. Presence of granuloma formation, transmural inflammation, lymphocytic infiltration. **(2)**
4. Endoscopic appearance:
   - Crohn's – inflammation is not continuous with presence of skip lesions. Cobblestone appearance of affected bowel
   - ulcerative colitis – inflammation is uniform, with thin walls and loss of vascular pattern.

Distribution:

- Crohn's – can be present from mouth to anus, commonly in terminal ileum
- ulcerative colitis – rectum always affected, affects large bowel only. **(3)**

5. Erythema nodosum, pyoderma gangrenosum, iritis/conjunctivitis/ episcleritis, large-joint arthritis, ankylosing spondylitis, apthous ulceration. **(1 mark for each, max 2 marks)**

6. Avoids long-term side effects of steroids in frequent relapses. **(1)**

7. Perianal abscess and fistulae, enteric fistulae, perforated bowel, small-bowel obstruction, colonic carcinoma, malnutrition. **(1 mark for each, max 2 marks)**

8. Antibody is directed against tumour necrosis factor, which is important in establishing inflammation and granuloma formation. **(1)**

Crohn's disease is a chronic inflammatory disease which can affect any part of the GI tract. Non-caseating granulomata are prominent on colonic histology from patients with Crohn's. Proposed causes include reaction to products of gut flora and a genetic predisposition. Crohn's is most commonly seen in white Caucasians, with onset in late teens or early twenties. Clinical features depend on the part of the bowel affected. Small-bowel Crohn's may present with abdominal pain, weight loss, diarrhoea and systemic symptoms of fever and malaise. Anal Crohn's may present as perianal abscesses, fistulae or fissures. Other symptoms may arise from small-bowel obstruction, intra-abdominal abscess or rarely peritonitis from free perforation. Extra-intestinal features include erythema nodosum, polyarthritis, anterior uveitis and pyoderma gangrenosum. Diagnosis can be made from abdominal CT scanning, colonoscopy or OGD. Small-bowel disease can be assessed by barium follow-through studies or capsule endoscopy. Medical treatment aims to induce remission with steroids, sometimes given parenterally in acute attacks, and long-term treatments are steroid-sparing, such as azathioprine or infliximab. Surgical interventions are to control septic complications or fistulas and are not curative.

# A²

1. Oesophagitis, Mallory-Weiss tear, oesophageal varices, peptic ulcers, gastritis/duodenitis, malignancy, bleeding disorders, angiodysplasia, aortic enteric fistula (rapidly fatal). **(2)**
2. NSAIDs, aspirin, cortocosteroids, anticoagulants, thrombolytics. **(2)**
3. Presence of melaena is evidence of large blood loss. **(1)**
4. Haemoglobin 13.0 – a fall in haemoglobin may not be seen very soon after bleeding, as the blood has not undergone haemodilution; urea 14.5, creatinine 67 – urea is raised out of proportion to creatinine. This is an indication of an upper gastrointestinal bleed. **(2)**
5. Urgent oesophagogastroduodenoscopy. **(1)**
6. Proton pump inhibitors. **(1)**
7. Liver cirrhosis. **(1)**
8. Venous portal hypertension. **(1)**
9. Superior rectal vein shunts cause haemorrhoids; paraumbilical vein shunts cause caput medusae. **(1 mark for each, max 2 marks)**
10. Adrenaline, sclerotherapy, banding of varices, argon plasma coagulation. **(1)**

Upper GI bleeding is a medical emergency, with many of the causes life-threatening. It may present with haematemesis, melaena and haemodynamic instability. In the presence of chronic liver disease, causes may be from peptic ulceration, gastritis or oesophageal varices. Haemodynamic instability should be promptly corrected with IV fluids and blood products to correct clotting abnormalities. Urgent endoscopy is the investigation of choice, and therapeutic measures such as variceal banding, sclerotherapy or argon plasma coagulation can be undertaken. Medical therapy for variceal bleeding includes reducing splanchnic blood flow using terlipressin and β-blockers. Risk of rebleeding can be assessed by applying a Rockall score, which uses age, haemodynamic stability, comorbidity and diagnosis at endoscopy to risk-stratify patients. Once acute bleeding has been stopped, risk of rebleeding is high, so secondary banding can be undertaken to reduce this risk. Surgical procedures such as transjugular intrahepatic portosystemic shunts can reduce portal pressures and reduce the risk of rebleeding.

# A³

1. Gastro-oesophageal reflux disease, gastritis, oesophagitis, duodenitis, malignancy. **(2)**

2. Symptoms of anaemia, weight loss, anorexia, recently worsening symptoms, dysphagia, melaena or haematemesis. **(2)**

3. *H. pylori* infection, medications: NSAIDs/steroids, smoking, delayed gastric emptying, physiological stress, e.g. in ITU patients, hypercalcaemia, chronic renal failure. **(1 mark for each, max 2 marks)**

4. *H. pylori* bacteria produce urease to break down urea into ammonia and carbon dioxide. A radio isotope of carbon (C-13 or C-14) in the form of urea is ingested, and if urease is present it breaks down urea, and radioisotope carbon dioxide can be measured. **(2)**

5. Two separate antibiotics for at least 2 weeks, plus a proton pump inhibitor. **(2)**

6. Erect chest X-ray. **(1)**

7. Pneumoperitoneum is seen as free air under the diaphragm. **(1)**

8. Oesophagogastroduodenoscopy. **(1)**

9. Zollinger-Ellison syndrome: ectopic gastrin production usually from a pancreatic gastrinoma or part of MEN syndrome. **(2)**

Peptic ulcer disease is a common disorder linked to stomach bacteria called *Helicobacter pylori*. Symptoms may be vague and chronic, such as epigastric pain related to food, bloating and fullness. Alarming symptoms which should prompt urgent referral are anaemia, weight loss, progressive recent symptoms, melaena, dysphagia, abdominal mass and palpable supraclavicular node. In younger patients, testing for *H. pylori* and triple therapy with two antibiotics and proton pump inhibitors are effective at eradicating the bacteria and improving symptoms. Ulcers in the duodenum are commoner than gastric ulcers by a ratio of 4 : 1. Medications such as NSAIDs, aspirin and steroids greatly increase the risk of gastritis and ulcer disease. Upper GI endoscopy is the investigation of choice for patients with alarming symptoms listed above. Lifestyle changes are smoking cessation, weight loss, alcohol reduction and avoidance of exacerbating foods.

# A⁴

1. Excessive entry of gastric contents into the oesophagus through the gastro-oesophageal junction. **(1)**
2. Lying flat, stooping, straining, drugs, alcohol, obesity, food, hiatus hernia. **(2)**
3. Inhalation of small amounts of gastric contents. **(1)**
4. Weight loss, smoking cessation, reduce alcohol consumption, avoid large meals, avoid eating before bedtime, sleep on an incline. **(2)**
5. Benign stricture secondary to GORD, malignant stricture (oesophageal/gastric/pharyngeal), extrinsic pressure from lung cancer, mediastinal lymph nodes, retrosternal goitre, pharyngeal pouch, oesophagitis, bulbar palsy, myasthenia gravis. **(2)**
6. A change of lower oesophageal squamous epithelium into columnar epithelium, caused by recurrent damage from gastric contents refluxing into the oesophagus. **(2)**
7. Oesophageal pH manometry. **(1)**
8. This augments the high-pressure zone, giving more strength to the GOJ. **(1)**
9. Dysphagia from compression of the GOJ, dumping syndrome, achalasia. **(1)**

Gastro-oesophageal reflux disease is caused by dysfunction of the lower oesophageal sphincter, allowing gastric contents to spill into the lower oesophagus. Prolonged or excessive reflux may cause oesophagitis, strictures and Barrett's oesophagus. It is associated with smoking, alcohol, hiatus hernia, obesity, large meals and systemic sclerosis. Controlling some of these lifestyle factors can help symptoms greatly, as can avoiding hot drinks and eating more than 3 hours before bedtime. Symptoms include epigastric and retrosternal discomfort, which can be exacerbated by food, position and straining, belching, regurgitation and odynophagia. Dysphagia, weight loss, recurrent symptoms and advancing age should initiate a referral for upper GI endoscopy. Management includes simple antacids, alginates, proton pump inhibitors and prokinetic anti-emetics. Surgical treatment in severe disease involves wrapping the gastric fundus around the lower oesophageal sphincter to increase its tone.

# A⁵

1. Pre-hepatic – anything that causes haemolysis e.g. malaria, sickle-cell disease, thalassemia, G6PD deficiency, spherocytosis, Gilbert's syndrome, Crigler-Najjar syndrome; intrahepatic/ hepatocellular – viral hepatitis, paracetamol overdose, drugs (anti-TB, statins, valproate, halothane), alcoholic hepatitis, liver tumour (primary/secondary), sepsis, alcoholic hepatitis, poisonous fungi, alpha-1-antitrypsin, Budd-Chiari, autoimmune hepatitis, haemochromatosis; cholestatic/obstructive – CBD bile stones, pancreatic cancer, porta hepatis lymph node, primary biliary sclerosis, sclerosing cholangitis, flucloxacillin, COCP, anabolic steroids. (3)

2. Haemoglobin. Haemoglobin → haem + globin → porphyrin + $Fe^{2+}$ → bilirubin. (1)

3. Cholestasis/obstructive. (1)

4. Bilirubin that has conjugated with gluconuride in hepatocytes is water-soluble, so dissolves in the urine, making it dark. (1)

5. Ultrasound scan of the abdomen. (1)

6. Endoscopic retrograde cholangiopancreatography (ERCP) + stenting of the CBD. (1)

7. Adenocarcinoma → mucinous cystic adenoma → islet cell tumours. (1)

8. Epigastric pain, back pain, weight loss, epigastric mass, dyspepsia, pruritus, fatigue, hepatomegaly from metastases. (2)

9. Ca19-9. (1)

10. Increased susceptibility to infection, pruritus, liver dysfunction, acute renal failure, nutritional dysfunction. (1)

Jaundice is the yellow discolouration of the skin, sclera and mucosa due to abnormally high levels of bilirubin in the bloodstream. Jaundice is classified by its cause, namely prehepatic jaundice from increased red cell breakdown, intrahepatic due to hepatocellular dysfunction and post-hepatic due to obstruction of the biliary tree. Bilirubin is formed by the breakdown of haemoglobin and is conjugated with glucuronide in the liver to make it water-soluble. Post-hepatic (obstructive) jaundice can be due to obstructing gallstones, tumours in the pancreas or bile duct, lymph nodes or primary sclerosing cholangitis. Pancreatic cancer is a serious cause of obstructive jaundice, with an insidious onset of weight loss, epigastric pain and anorexia. Prognosis is poor due to a late presentation, which often makes surgical resection impossible or distant metastases are present. Treatment in these cases is palliative, with relief of obstructed bile ducts or chemotherapy. Diagnosis can be made from CT scanning or ERCP, with response to treatment being monitored by measurement of Ca19-9.

# A6

1. Hepatitic. **(1)**
2. Hepatitis A – faecal-oral spread; hepatitis B – blood-borne. **(2)**
3. IV drug users and their sexual partners, sex workers, healthcare workers, haemophiliacs, close contacts of carriers or new cases. **(2)**
4. Past infection. **(1)**
5. Fulminant hepatic failure, cholestasis, chronic hepatitis, cirrhosis, hepatocellular cancer, glomerulonephritis, cryoglobulinaemia. **(2)**
6. Bleed the site and wash thoroughly, urgently attend A&E or occupational health for advice and possibly post-exposure prophylaxis. **(1)**
7. HIV, hepatitis C, hepatitis D. **(1 mark for each, max 2 marks)**

Viral hepatitis is a common cause of hepatocellular jaundice. Hepatitis A is spread by the faecal-oral route and is often transient and self-limiting; there is currently a vaccine available for all those travelling to affected areas. Hepatitis B and C are both blood-borne viruses, and therefore risk factors all involve inoculation of infected blood. They include sexual intercourse, blood transfusions or injections using infected needles. At-risk groups include intravenous drug users, sex workers, healthcare workers and haemophiliacs. Hepatitis B is a DNA virus that is endemic in the Far East, Africa and the Mediterranean. Acute infection symptoms include fever, malaise, anorexia, arthralgia, jaundice and hepatosplenomegaly. Complications include chronic carriage with cirrhosis, chronic hepatitis and an increased risk of hepatocellular carcinoma. Treatment is mainly supportive where interferon alpha and lamivudine have a role. Population strategies include widespread vaccination of high-risk groups using a suspension of hepatitis B surface antigen (HbSAg).

# A⁷

1. Alcohol abuse. **(1)**
2. An inherited cause of cirrhosis: haemochromatosis, Wilson's disease, alpha-1-antitrypsin deficiency.

   An acquired cause of cirrhosis: chronic alcohol abuse, chronic viral hepatitis, autoimmune hepatitis, primary biliary cirrhosis, venous obstruction, idiopathic. **(1 mark for each, max 2 marks)**
3. Leuconychia, clubbing, palmar erythema, Dupuytren's contracture, spider naevi, gynaecomastia, atrophic testes, hepatosplenomegaly, ascites. **(1 mark for each, max 2 marks)**
4. Albumin or INR/PT (indirectly assesses synthesis of clotting factors). **(1 mark for each, max 2 marks)**
5. Coagulopathy, encephalopathy, hypoalbuminaemia, sepsis, spontaneous bacterial peritonitis, hypoglycaemia, ascites, oesophageal varices. **(1 mark for each, max 2 marks)**
6. Fluid restriction, low-sodium diet/fluids, diuretics, abdominal paracentesis (ascitic drainage), albumin infusion. **(1 mark for each, max 2 marks)**
7. White cell count, MC&S, cytology, albumin/LDH/glucose. **(1 mark for each, max 2 marks)**
8. Increasing bowel transit reduces the number of nitrogen-producing bacteria in the gut, which contributes to hepatic encephalopathy. **(1)**
9. Liver transplantation. **(1)**

Liver cirrhosis is chronic irreversible liver damage with loss of hepatic cellular architecture. Macroscopically, the liver looks shrunken, scarred and nodular. The commonest cause in the UK is long-term alcohol abuse. Where it is endemic chronic hepatitis B or C, infection is also a common cause. There are many signs of chronic liver disease, such as clubbing, leuconychia, palmar erythema, spider naevi and ascites. Severe liver dysfunction results in coagulopathy, encephalopathy, hypoalbuminaemia, susceptibility to sepsis, hypoglycaemia and peritonitis. When the cause is in doubt, investigations include ultrasound and duplex scanning, ferritin, total iron-binding capacity, hepatitis serology, autoantibodies, alpha fetoprotein, caeruloplasmin and alpha-1-antitrypsin. Management aims to reduce deterioration with low-salt diets to avoid ascites, alcohol abstinence and avoiding hepatotoxic medications and medications metabolised in the liver as well as opiates and sedatives. Definitive treatment depends on the cause; complications such as ascites should be treated with diuretics and drainage. Spontaneous bacterial peritonitis should be urgently treated with IV antibiotics according to local protocol.

# A⁸

1. Crohn's disease, chronic pancreatitis, cystic fibrosis, short bowel syndrome, dumping syndrome, tropical sprue. **(1 mark for each, max 2 marks)**

2. Diarrhoea/steatorrhoea, nausea and vomiting, fatigue, iron-deficiency anaemia, osteomalacia, failure to thrive, infertility, IgA deficiency, rash (dermatitis herpetiformis). **(1 mark for each, max 2 marks)**

3. Autoimmune disease (where gluten proteins are modified by and presented to T cells which cause inflammation of the small bowel tissue). **(1)**

4. Wheat. **(1)**

5. Tissue transglutaminase, full blood count, iron studies, haematinics, bone profile. **(1)**

6. Severe malabsorption can cause deficiency in proteins such as IgA. **(1)**

7. Villous atrophy, increased intraepithelial lymphocytes, hypoplasia of small-bowel architecture, proliferation of crypts of Lieberkuhn. **(1)**

8. Complete gluten-free diet. **(1)**

9. Type 1 diabetes, thyroid disease, microscopic colitis. **(1 mark for each, max 2 marks)**

10. GI T-cell lymphoma, Gastric, Oesophageal. **(1 mark for each, max 2 marks)**

Coeliac disease is a T-cell-mediated autoimmune disease affecting the small bowel in which prolamin found in rye, barley and wheat causes loss of villous architecture, which leads to malabsorption. It is associated with HLA-DQ2 and is commoner in northern European populations. Symptoms include abdominal pain, weight loss, weakness and steatorrhoea. Iron-deficiency anaemia may also be present. Time to diagnosis may be delayed, so a high index of suspicion is important. Blood investigations include antibodies to alpha-gliadin, tissue transglutaminase and endomysial. Gold-standard diagnosis is duodenal biopsies, which reveal villous atrophy. The best treatment is complete removal of gluten from the diet, which should be maintained for life. Gluten-free food is available on prescription, and patients should be educated on the foods to avoid. Complications include T cell lymphoma, increased risk of malignancy and effects of malnutrition.

# A⁹

1. Drug-induced:
   - opiate use
   - anticholinergic medication
   - iron.

   Mechanical:
   - colorectal cancer
   - stricture (e.g. Crohn's)
   - pelvic mass (e.g. gynaecological malignancy).

   Lifestyle:
   - dehydration
   - immobility
   - poor diet
   - poor environment or toilet facilities. **(1 mark for each group, max 3 marks)**

2. Abdominal pain which is relieved by defacation, alternating constipation and diarrhoea, bloating, mucous per rectum, tenesmus, reflux, epigastric pain. **(2)**

3. Full blood count: look for anaemia.

   Thyroid function tests: hypothyroidism can cause constipation and hyperthyroidism can cause diarrhoea.

   Sigmoidoscopy: look for rectal cause of symptoms, such as polyps, tumours or evidence of inflammatory bowel disease. **(1 mark for each, max 3 marks)**

4. Depression, stress disorder, anxiety. **(1)**

5. Colonoscopy **(1)** in order to investigate right side of colon. Right-sided colonic tumours may present as unexplained iron-deficiency anaemia. **(1)**

6. Neoplastic polyps, ulcerative colitis, Crohn's disease, familial adenomatous polyps, hereditary non-polyposis colorectal carcinoma (HNPCC), low-fibre diet. **(1 mark for each, max 2 marks)**

7. Liver, lung, bone, local invasion, lymphatic spread. **(1)**

Irritable bowel syndrome is a primarily functional disorder which covers a large number of intestinal symptoms and classically was a diagnosis of exclusion. Whilst aetiology is not certain, gastrointestinal motility and visceral perception problems are mooted as possibilities. Commoner in young females, symptoms include left-sided or central abdominal pain, bloating, changing bowel habit, nausea and symptoms of reflux. Symptoms may be cyclical with menstruation or related to psychological stressors. Treatment is symptomatic and many specialties may be involved. Constipation can be treated with increased dietary fibre with ispaghul husk, whilst diarrhoea can be treated with bulking agents and loperamide. Antispasmodics such as mebeverine can be used if colicky pain or spasm is prominent. Exclusion diets can help if lactose intolerance is involved. Psychological therapy can help with concurrent stress and depression. It is important however to screen for worrying symptoms such as weight loss and per rectal bleeding that may have a serious cause.

# A¹⁰

1. *Shigella, Campylobacter, E. coli, C. difficile, Salmonella, Yersinia, Staphylococcus, Vibrio cholerae.* **(1 mark for each, max 2 marks)**

2. Rotavirus, norovirus, adenovirus, astrovirus. **(1)**

3. Oral or IV fluid rehydration, anti-emetics for vomiting, analgesia for abdominal pain. **(1 mark for each, max 3 marks)**

4. *C. difficile*-associated diarrhoea/pseudomembranous colitis. **(1)**

5. Metronidazole, oral vancomycin. **(2)**

6. Barrier nursing, isolation of patient(s), adequate hand-washing, personal protective measures, (e.g. gloves, masks, aprons), reduce number of contacts with patient. **(1 mark for each, max 2 marks)**

Gastroenteritis is an acute infection of the GI tract which results in acute-onset diarrhoea with vomiting and abdominal pain. In the developing world, without access to clean water and medical attention, gastroenteritis is a leading cause of mortality. Complications arise from dehydration, and treatment is directed to correcting this and alleviating symptoms.

Antibiotics should only be given if systemically unwell, immune-compromised or a known sensitive organism has been cultured. Most acute causes are due to viruses, although stool samples should be sent for bacterial and protozoal infection. If a food source is most likely, it is a notifiable disease in the UK, and contact tracing is encouraged to prevent outbreaks. Some virulent strains of bacteria such as *E. coli* O157 can cause outbreaks of typhoid-like symptoms and can be haemorrhagic with development of haemolytic uraemic syndrome.

# Neurology

## A¹

1. Arterial. **(1)**
2. Berry or saccular aneurysms. **(1)**
3. Polycystic kidney disease, Ehlers–Danlos syndrome, coarctation of the aorta. **(1)**
4. Vomiting, collapse, seizures, coma, visual disturbance/photophobia, focal neurological signs, e.g. hemiplegia, dysphasia (due to haematoma). **(½ a mark each, max 2 marks)**
5. Kernig's sign demonstrates meningeal irritation. **(1)** The hip and knee is bent to 90 degrees, it is a positive if pain is caused by straightening the knee. **(1)**
6. CT head – blood appears white; this will be mixed in with the CSF. This will lie within the interhemispheric fissure, basal cisterns and ventricles. **(2)**
7. Lumbar puncture, xanthochromia. **(2)**

Subarachnoid haemorrhage should be suspected for any patient with sudden onset of severe headache, often described as the 'first and worst', 'thunderclap' or 'being hit by a baseball bat'. The CT head can be normal in a small bleed, so if there is clinical suspicion, a lumbar puncture should also be performed. The sample of CSF should be analysed for xanthochromia, a breakdown product from bilirubin. Blood may be present in the CSF if blood made its way into the sample during the lumbar puncture – a 'traumatic tap'.

## A²

1. 11. **(1)**
2. Lucid interval. **(1)**
3. Parietal bone, temporal bone, sphenoid bone, frontal bone. **(½ a mark for each, max 2 marks)**
4. Arterial. **(1)**
5. Venous. **(1)**

6. An extradural haematoma is often described as lens-shaped or biconvex. A subdural haematoma is described as being crescent-shaped. **(1 mark for each, max 2 marks)**
7. Midline shift, compression of the ventricles. **(2)**

Extradural haematomas often result from a skull fracture leading to a laceration to the middle meningeal artery. The pterion is relevant as the anterior division of the middle meningeal artery runs underneath it. The bleed into the fixed space causes a rise in intracranial pressure, with subsequent midline shift and herniation. Ultimately, evacuation and ligation of the bleeding vessel is needed.

# A³

1. Diabetes, heart disease (e.g. atrial fibrillation, valvular), peripheral vascular disease, previous TIA, polycythaemia rubra vera, carotid artery disease, hyperlipidaemia, clotting disorders, combined oral contraceptive pill, excess alcohol. **(½ a mark for each, max 2 marks)**
2. A stroke lasts over 24 hours or leads to death within 24 hours. **(1)**
3. Hemiplegia. **(1)**
4. Left-sided sensory loss, dysphasia, homonymous hemianopia. **(1 mark for each, max 2 marks)**
5. Carotid artery atherosclerosis **(1)**, carotid endarterectomy can be offered for severe stenosis. **(1)**
6. Admission to stroke unit, swallow assessment, physiotherapy, skin care. **(1 mark for each, max 2 marks)**

A stroke is a clinical syndrome of a presumed vascular territory that lasts for over 24 hours or leads to death before this. A majority of strokes are caused by ischaemic events. It is important to fully explain what has happened to the patient, family and carers. Primary prevention is the key and consists of controlling risk factors. These include lowering BP, stopping smoking, well-controlled diabetes, reducing cholesterol and lipids, improving diet and exercise.

# A⁴

1. Transient occurrence of intermittent, abnormal electrical activity of part of the brain. This tends to be stereotyped and often manifests itself as seizures. **(1)**
2. An aura is part of the seizure and often precedes other manifestations. It is a disturbance of a sensation, often a strange feeling, smell, taste or flashing lights. **(1)**
3. Temporary weakness following a seizure – usually of affected limb(s). **(1)**
4. Generalised tonic-clonic epilepsy. **(1)**
5. Partial seizure: features focal to one hemisphere, for example, a motor region (can be elementary symptoms with consciousness unimpaired or complex with consciousness impaired).

   Partial seizure with secondary generalization: seizure starts focally then spreads, causing a generalised seizure.

   Absence seizure: a generalised seizure, brief pauses, for example, stops talking for a period then continues from where they stopped.

   Atonic: patient becomes flaccid. **(1 mark for each, max 2 marks)**
6. Uraemia, hypoglycaemia, hyponatraemia, hypernatraemia, hypocalcaemia, anoxia, water intoxification. **(2)**
7. Nasopharyngeal airway. **(1)**
8. Roll the patient into the recovery position and move any items away from him that could cause harm. Place a pillow under his head. Give oxygen. Call for senior help. Give IV bolus of benzodiazepine in accordance with trust policy (e.g. diazepam or lorazepam), *do not* try to place anything in his mouth, including suction. **(½ a mark for each, max 2 marks)**

Epilepsy may be due to a structural brain abnormality, metabolic abnormalities, drugs or alcohol (or withdrawal) or hypoxia; however, most are idiopathic. A patient is said to be in status epilepticus if the seizure lasts > 30 minutes or has repeated seizures without regaining consciousness between. Mortality and brain damage increases with the length of the seizure, and therefore you should be aiming to terminate seizure activity lasting over a few minutes as quickly as possible.

# A⁵

1. Bitemporal hemianopia. **(1)**
2. Optic chiasm. **(1)**
3. Pituitary gland **(1)**, likely to be a non-functioning adenoma as no endocrine symptoms are apparent. **(1)**
4. Medial. **(1)**
5. Visual acuity, visual fields, fundoscopy, pupillary light response (direct and indirect), pupillary accommodation, eye movements. **(½ a mark for each, max 3 marks)**
6. Unilateral damage to the optic radiation or visual cortex. **(2)**

Bitemporal hemianopia usually results from damage at the optic chiasm where the nasal (medial) retinal nerve fibres cross to the contralateral side. The nasal retinal field visualises the temporal (lateral) visual field. This condition can arise from compression from an enlarged pituitary gland. These can be functioning or non-functioning tumours. Functioning tumours will give rise to endocrine abnormalities, for example, acromegaly, hyperprolactinaemia, Cushing's disease, thyrotoxicosis.

# A⁶

1. Joint-position sense and pressure. **(2)**
2. Posteriorly. **(1)**
3. Within the medulla. **(1)**
4. Pain, temperature (crude touch). **(1 mark for each, max 2 marks)**
5. Anterior portion. **(1)**
6. Ischaemia from anterior spinal artery occlusion. **(1)**
7. Ipsilateral (left-sided) spastic paralysis and loss of vibration and proprioception **(1)** and contralateral loss of pain and temperature sensation. **(1)**

Good anatomical knowledge of where spinal tracts run within the spinal cord and where they decussate is crucial to establishing what has been affected in any patient with a spinal pathology. Pain and temperature are carried by the spinothalamic tract and joint position and pressure sensation by the dorsal columns. The corticospinal tracts carry the motor neurones. Most motor neurones (around 80%) will cross over to the contralateral side in the medulla oblongata.

# A⁷

1. Dura mater, arachnoid mater, pia mater. (**1 mark each**)
2. *Streptococcus pneumoniae, Neisseria meningitidis.* (**1 mark each**)
3. Pain and resistance on knee extension with the hips fully flexed. (**1**)
4. Meningococcal septicaemia (NB: not meningitis). (**1**)
5. To rule out raised intracranial pressure. (**1**)
6. Benzylpenicillin. (**1**)
7. Cephalosporins (third generation – cefotaxime, ceftriaxone). (**1**)

Meningitis is inflammation of the meninges of the brain. It is often viral in origin, but due to the significant morbidity and mortality associated with bacterial meningitis, all cases should be treated as bacterial until proven otherwise. Infants, young children and the elderly are the most susceptible age groups. Patients present with fever, headache, photophobia, neck stiffness or altered mental consciousness, but in the high-risk age groups mentioned above, patients may present with non-specific symptoms and signs, so a high index of suspicion is required. It is important to understand that a petechial rash is seen in meningococcal septicaemia and is not in itself a sign of meningitis. Lumbar puncture is essential, but CT head scans should be performed if there are concerns regarding raised intracranial pressure. Early antibiotic therapy is important to reduce the morbidity and mortality, and empirical antibiotics should be commenced prior to knowing culture results. Supportive therapy such as analgesia antipyretics and hydration is also required. It is important to remember that meningitis is a notifiable disease.

# A⁸

1. Median nerve. (**1**)
2. Two lateral lumbricals, opponens pollicis, abductor pollicis brevis, flexor pollicis brevis. (**½ a mark each**)
3. Wrist flexion for a maximum of 60 seconds elicits paraesthesia in the median nerve distribution. (**1**)
4. Tapping over the median nerve at the wrist elicits paraesthesia in the median nerve distribution. (**1**)

5. Pregnancy, menopause, oral contraceptive pill, obesity, trauma, diabetes mellitus, hypothyroidism, rheumatoid arthritis, acromegaly, amyloidosis, dialysis, repetitive activities, local compression (e.g. lipoma, ganglion). **(2)**
6. Electroneurography, electromyography, ultrasonography, MRI scan. **(1)**
7. Splinting, local corticosteroid injection, carpal tunnel release surgery. **(2)**

The carpal tunnel is the space between the flexor retinaculum and the underlying carpal bones, and through it run the median nerve and the tendons of the flexor digitorum profundus, flexor digitorum superficialis and flexor pollicis longus. An increase in pressure within this closed space may lead to compression of the median nerve, giving rise to carpal tunnel syndrome. The clinical features include numbness, paraesthesia and pain in the median nerve distribution which are often worse at night, weakness of the 'LOAF' muscles supplied by the median nerve and wasting of the thenar eminence. Phalen's and Tinel's tests are performed as part of the physical examination, and if positive increase the suspicion of carpal tunnel syndrome. Neurophysiological studies may show a slowing of conduction of the nerve impulse across the carpal tunnel. The role of imaging to aid diagnosis remains unclear.

## A⁹

1. Bradykinesia, rigidity, postural instability. **(2)**
2. Dopamine. **(1)**
3. Lewy bodies. **(1)**
4. Peripheral dopa-decarboxylase inhibitor, as it reduces peripheral breakdown, leading to a decreased dose of levodopa required for symptom control and therefore a reduced risk of side effects. **(2)**
5. On-off fluctuations, dyskinesias, weaning off phenomenon. **(2)**
6. Dopamine agonists, monoamine oxidase B-inhibitors, catechol-O-methyl transferase inhibitors, anticholinergics, amantadine, surgery. **(2)**

Parkinson's disease is caused by degeneration of the dopaminergic neurones in the substantia nigra of the basal ganglia. The pathological finding is of Lewy bodies in this area. The main features of Parkinson's disease are tremor, bradykinesia, rigidity and postural instability. Depression, psychosis and dementia may occur in these patients. The diagnosis is usually made on clinical findings, but may be aided by CT, MRI or PET scans. In addition to managing the clinical features of Parkinson's disease with medications such as levodopa, it is important to consider the additional support these patients will require, so involvement of a multidisciplinary team including doctors, physiotherapists, occupational therapists and speech and language therapists is essential. It is important to note that Parkinson's disease is not the only condition to give rise to Parkinsonism – the clinical features listed above. Other causes include neuroleptic medications, multiple system atrophy and progressive supranuclear palsy.

## A¹⁰

1. Morning. **(1)**
2. Lying down, coughing, bending. **(1)**
3. Vomiting, papilloedema, seizures, focal neurology, decreased conscious level. **(2)**
4. Neoplasm, haematoma, abscess, granuloma, aneurysm. **(2)**
5. Frontal lobe. **(1)**
6. CT scan. **(1)**
7. Mannitol, dexamethasone. **(2)**

Commonly, space-occupying lesions within the cranial cavity are due to neoplasms. They may present with features of raised intracranial pressure, such as headaches and vomiting, or alternatively with focal neurological features. CT scans should be performed in the A&E department if raised intracranial pressure is suspected to rule out life-threatening causes. MRI is better at defining soft tissue lesions but is not commonly available in the acute setting. Cases of space-occupying lesions should be discussed with neurosurgeons to determine if surgical intervention is appropriate.

# General surgery

1. Anorexia, nausea, vomiting, fever, constipation, diarrhoea. **(2)**
2. Irritation of the visceral peritoneum by the inflamed appendix is felt in the T10 dermatome, which corresponds to the periumbilical region. This is because the visceral peritoneum has no somatic innervation, so the brain perceives visceral signals as being from the same dermatome as where the visceral signals enter the spinal cord. As the appendix is found in the midgut, the corresponding dermatome is T10. **(1)**
3. As the disease progresses, the parietal peritoneum becomes affected. As this receives somatic innervations, the pain is well localised to the area of inflammation. **(1)**
4. Rovsing's sign is pain felt in the right iliac fossa when the left iliac fossa is palpated. **(1)**
5. The differential for appendicitis is wide. It comprises ectopic pregnancy, torsion/rupture of ovarian cyst, salpingitis, UTI, renal stone, testicular torsion, GI obstruction, constipation, strangulated hernia, Crohn's disease, gastroenteritis, mesenteric adenitis, Meckel's diverticulum and intussusception. **(2)**
6. Appendicectomy. **(1)**
7. Perforation, appendix mass (omentum and small bowel adhere to appendix), abscess, sepsis, paralytic ileus, intestinal obstruction. **(2)**

Acute appendicitis is the commonest cause of an acute abdomen in the UK. The lumen of the appendix becomes obstructed, commonly by faecoliths or lymphoid hyperplasia, leading to stasis of the contents of the appendix and subsequently invasion of the appendix wall by gut flora, leading to inflammation. The typical pattern of progression is periumbilical pain migrating to the right iliac fossa, as described above. The diagnosis is essentially clinical, but a raised white cell count, neutrophil count and CRP will increase suspicion of appendicitis. A pregnancy test should always be performed in a woman of childbearing age to rule out an ectopic pregnancy. Imaging is only reserved for cases where the diagnosis is unclear and the modalities of choice are USS or CT scan. Prompt appendicectomy should be performed once the diagnosis is made.

## A²

1. An outpouching of mucosa through the muscle wall. **(1)**
2. Sigmoid colon, as in this part of the bowel the majority of water has been reabsorbed from the faeces, leading to high intraluminal pressures. **(1)**
3. Diverticulosis – the presence of diverticula in the GI tract; diverticular disease – symptomatic diverticula; diverticulitis – inflammation of diverticula. **(1 mark for each)**
4. FBC, CRP, blood cultures, CXR, AXR, CT scan, USS. **(2)**

   (NB: barium enemas/endoscopy should be avoided in the acute phase due to the risk of perforation.)
5. Analgesia, antibiotics, adequate hydration. **(1)**
6. Perforation, bleeding, abscess, strictures, fistulas. **(2)**

It is important to distinguish between diverticulosis, diverticular disease and diverticulitis. Diverticulosis is asymptomatic. Diverticular disease causes such symptoms as lower abdominal pain, bloating, constipation and rectal bleeding. Diverticulitis is accompanied by signs of inflammation, such as fever, tachycardia and peritonism, in addition to raised inflammatory markers. When diverticulitis is diagnosed, CXRs and AXRs may be performed to rule out such complications as perforation and obstruction. USS may demonstrate collections and free fluid, but CT scan is a more accurate test. The majority of diverticulitis cases will respond to conservative management, but occasionally surgical resection of the affected segment of bowel is required. Following the acute phase, barium enemas or endoscopy (sigmoidoscopy/colonoscopy) can be performed for further assessment.

## A³

1. The protrusion of a structure through the wall of cavity in which it is usually contained. **(1)**
2. The neck of an inguinal hernia appears superior and medial to the pubic tubercle. The neck of a femoral hernia appears inferior and lateral to it. **(1)**

3. Indirect inguinal hernias occur lateral to the inferior epigastric vessels; direct inguinal hernias occur medial to these vessels. **(1)**

4. During foetal development, the testes descend from the posterior abdominal wall into the scrotum following the processus vaginalis via an attachment called the gubernaculums. If the connection to the peritoneal cavity fails to close, then a patent processus vaginalis is present through which indirect inguinal hernias can occur. **(1 mark for each)**

5. Prematurity, male sex, chronic cough, constipation, obesity, heavy lifting, other physical activity, e.g. sports. **(2)**

6. An obstructed inguinal hernia is one through which contents of the GI tract cannot pass. A strangulated inguinal hernia implies ischaemia of the portion of bowel affected. **(1)**

7. Recurrence, wound site infection, mesh infection, hydrocoele, intestinal damage, bladder damage, spermatic cord damage, testicular infarction secondary to blood vessel damage. **(2)**

Inguinal hernias are the commonest form of hernia. Indirect hernias pass through the internal inguinal ring into the inguinal canal, and if large enough, through the external inguinal ring into the scrotum. Direct inguinal hernias protrude directly through the abdominal wall into the inguinal canal. Indirect hernias comprise 80% of inguinal hernias, and direct hernias make up the remaining 20%. These hernias may be repaired electively unless the hernia becomes incarcerated, obstructed or strangulated, when the repair must be done as an emergency.

# A⁴

1. Dentate line. **(1)**
2. Anal itching, mucous, rectal fullness, pain, soiling. **(2)**
3. FBC, proctoscopy, sigmoidoscopy. **(2)**
4. Increase fluid intake, increase fibre intake, analgesia, bed rest, topical therapies (anaesthetics/corticosteroids). **(2)**
5. Rubber band ligation, sclerotherapy, cryotherapy, photocoagulation, haemorrhoidectomy, stapled haemorrhoidopexy, transanal haemorrhoidal dearterialisation. **(2)**
6. Ulceration, stricture, thrombosis, infection, anaemia, skin tags. **(1)**

Haemorrhoids are engorged vascular cushions in the anal canal. Viewed in the lithotomy position, they lie in the 3, 7 and 11 o'clock positions.

They are not varicose veins, and because the bleeding occurs from capillaries it is bright red in colour. If they occur above the dentate line, they are known as internal haemorrhoids, and below they are known as external haemorrhoids. As internal haemorrhoids arise above the dentate line, the overlying mucosa receives no somatic innervations, so they are painless unless they become prolapsed and thrombosed. The main reason for haemorrhoids occurring is constipation with prolonged straining. Other factors implicated include pregnancy, childbirth, chronic cough, heavy lifting and ascites. Conservative management aims to relieve pain and treat and prevent constipation. There are several outpatient procedures that may be used, such as rubber band ligation, sclerotherapy, cryotherapy and photocoagulation, but failure of these techniques may necessitate an operative procedure.

# A5

1. Foregut – celiac trunk; midgut – superior mesenteric artery; hindgut – inferior mesenteric artery. **(1 mark for each)**
2. Metabolic acidosis. **(1)**
3. Raised WCC, raised lactate, raised Hb (due to haemoconcentration), raised amylase. **(2)**
4. Angiography. **(1)**
5. Resection of necrotic bowel, revascularisation. **(2)**
6. Aggressive fluid resuscitation, antibiotics, heparin, analgesia. **(1)**

Acute mesenteric ischaemia is commonly due to arterial thrombosis, arterial embolism, venous thrombosis or non-occlusive ischaemia (often due to poor cardiac output). The pathogenesis involves reduced blood flow to the intestines, bacterial translocation across the dying intestinal wall and systemic inflammatory response syndrome. The classic presentation is of acute severe abdominal pain with minimal or no abdominal signs. The degree of pain is out of keeping with the clinical findings. Blood tests may often reveal a metabolic acidosis with a raised white cell count. AXRs are often non-specific in the early phase, CT scanning is often used to assist in the diagnosis, but angiography remains the gold standard. Aggressive fluid resuscitation, antibiotics and heparin are important in the initial management. Early surgical revascularisation with the removal of necrotic bowel remains the treatment of choice, but thrombolytics at the time of angiography and embolectomy may also have a role. Prognosis of acute mesenteric ischaemia is poor, especially if diagnosis is not made early.

## A⁶

1. Left kidney, left adrenal gland, splenic flexure of the colon (also transverse and descending accepted), pancreas, stomach, left lobe of liver, lung. **(2)**
2. The red pulp acts as the filter and destroys defunct red blood cells. **(1)**
3. The white pulp is lymphoid tissue which acts as part of the body's immune system. **(1)**
4. Spontaneous rupture, hypersplenism, neoplasia, cysts, splenic abscess. **(2)**
5. Encapsulated bacteria. **(1)**
6. Lifelong prophylactic antibiotics (penicillin V or erythromycin), vaccinations (pneumococcal, meningococcal, influenza, *Haemophilus influenzae* b). **(2)**
7. Red blood cells in which the nuclear remnant is still seen. **(1)**

The spleen has two main functions: to filter deformed red blood cells out of the circulation and as part of the body's immune system. Splenectomies may be a planned procedure, but in certain situations such as trauma they may be done as emergencies. Immediate postoperative complications include thrombocytosis and infection. Due to their lifelong risk of infection due to encapsulated organisms, patients are commenced on antibiotic prophylaxis and are advised regarding the need for immunisations. Patients should be advised to wear alert bracelets and carry cards to alert healthcare professionals to their risk of overwhelming infection.

## A⁷

1. Alcohol. **(1)**
2. Gallstones, alcohol, trauma, steroids, mumps, autoimmune, scorpion sting, hyperlipidaemia, hypothermia, hypercalcaemia, ERCP, drugs. **(½ a mark for each, max 2 marks)**
3. Amylase, commonly used but can be normal even in severe pancreatitis! Serum lipase is more sensitive. **(1)**
4. Shock, ARDS, sepsis, DIC, renal failure. **(2)**
5. Pancreatic pseudocyst, pancreatic necrosis, abscess, thrombosis of splenic/duodenal arteries, chronic pancreatitis. **(2)**

6. Fluid management, analgesia, NG tube, intensive care. **(1 mark for each, max 2 marks)**

There are many causes of pancreatitis, with the main ones being alcohol and gallstones. The inflammation of the pancreas also affects the surrounding tissues. Third-space sequestration needs aggressive fluid management to counterbalance it. Patients may appear well even in severe disease and can deteriorate quickly. Complex imaging such as CT is used to assess severity and abdominal ultrasound if gallstones are suspected.

# A8

1. Constipation (may not be absolute), vomiting, colicky abdominal pain, distension. **(2)**
2. Small-bowel obstruction (any two of the following): pain is higher in the abdomen as it is a midgut structure, vomiting occurs earlier and abdominal distension is less. **(2)**
3. Constipation, adhesions, hernias, tumour, diverticulitis. **(2)**
4. Absence of bowel sounds indicates an ileus. Tinkling bowel sounds supports a mechanical obstruction. **(1)**
5. Abdominal X-ray. **(1)**
6. Bowel rest – 'drip and suck'. The patient should be made nil by mouth and a nasogastric tube should be passed to rest the bowel from the gastric contents produced each day. Intravenous fluids should be started to adequately rehydrate the patient. **(2)**

It is important to establish whether there is a bowel strangulation causing the bowel obstruction, as this will need emergency surgery. The patient will present more unwell, there is sharper, constant abdominal pain and signs of peritonism. On an abdominal X-ray, the small bowel can be distinguished from the large bowel as it contains valvuli conniventes (lines across the lumen), appears 'grey' as is mixture of free gas and liquid, is more central in the abdomen and its diameter is usually around 2.5 cm. The large bowel contains haustra, which do not cross the lumen, it tends to lie more peripherally on the abdominal film and appears darker due to the gas. The colon is around 5 cm wide and 10 cm at the caecum.

# A⁹

1. Bile salts, bile pigments, cholesterol, phospholipid, electrolytes, water. **(2)**
2. Pigment stones, cholesterol stones, mixed stones. **(2)**
3. Fair (Caucasian), forty, fertile, fat, female. **(2)**
4. Two fingers are laid in the right upper quadrant and the patient is asked to breathe in; this has to cause pain and stop the patient breathing in fully. **(1)** It is positive if the test is repeated in the left upper quadrant and does not cause pain. **(1)**
5. Biliary ultrasound. **(1)**
6. Nil by mouth, intravenous fluids, analgesia, antibiotics. **(1)**

Biliary colic occurs when gallstones become symptomatic. Acute cholecystitis follows a stone impaction which causes local inflammation. Inflammatory markers will be raised, and on billiary ultrasound a thick-walled, shrunken gall bladder may be found with a common bile duct over 7 mm in diameter. If the gallstones block the outflow from the common hepatic duct, an obstructive jaundice can also develop. A cholecystectomy can be undertaken within 72 hours or will be performed at a later date when the inflammation has resolved at around 6–12 weeks.

# A¹⁰

1. Right, left, caudate, quadrate. **(2)**
2. Falciform ligament. **(1)**
3. GI tract, breast, lung, uterus. **(2)**
4. Viral hepatitis, cirrhosis (alcohol, haemchromatosis, primary biliary cirrhosis), aflatoxin, parasites, steroids, combined oral contraceptive pill. **(3)**
5. Alpha-fetoprotein. **(1)**

Tumours in the liver are usually secondary to metastatic tumours. Resection can be undertaken for small, solitary metastasis. Liver biopsy is crucial for diagnosis. Primary hepatic tumours can be benign or malignant. Haemangiomas and adenomas are common benign liver tumours.

# Urology

## A¹

1. Urinary tract infection, benign prostatic hyperplasia, constipation, medications (anticholinergic, opiates, antidepressants), pelvic nerve damage, post-anaesthesia, alcohol. (½ **a mark for each, max 2 marks)**

2. Peripheral nervous system (assess lower limbs for cauda equina compression). **(1)**

3. Document residual volume, take specimen for CSU, retract foreskin over glans penis. **(1 mark for each, max 2 marks)**

4. Full blood count, MSU, renal USS (if U&E elevated). NB: PSA is contentious; would be elevated in retention anyway. (½ **a mark for each, max 1 mark)**

5. Insulin 15 units + dextrose 50 ml 50%, 10% calcium gluconate, calcium resonium, salbutamol nebulisers. (½ **a mark for each, max 2 marks)**

6. Acute: chronic retention is more likely to hold higher volumes, e.g. 1.5 L+ and be painless. **(1)**

7. Post-obstructive diuresis: hourly urine output monitoring with replacement of losses with IV fluids. **(2)**

8. Tamsulosin: alpha-1 (a preferential to b) receptor antagonist. Relaxes prostatic smooth muscle. Finasteride: anti-androgen 5-alpha reductase inhibitor. Inhibits conversion of testosterone to dihydrotestosterone, which is a more potent androgen in prostatic tissue. **(1 mark for drug and 1 mark for mechanism, max 4 marks)**

Acute urinary retention is the painful inability to pass urine. It is frequently due to benign or malignant prostatic disease. Acute urinary retention should be treated as a medical emergency and with analgesia and prompt drainage of the bladder. Large volumes may be present should it be an acute or chronic problem. Chronic retention sometimes presents as incontinence due to overflow pressure. Acute urinary retention is an important and easily treatable cause of acute kidney injury. Inability to pass a catheter should prompt the clinical team to seek urological advice in order to drain urine, possibly by a suprapubic catheter. Medical treatment for benign prostatic hyperplasia includes alpha-1 adrenoceptor blockers and anti-androgens. Surgical techniques include minimal access surgery, such as transurethral resection of the prostate. These come with risks of long-term incontinence and erectile dysfunction.

# A²

1. Urinary tract infection, renal tract trauma, renal tract tumour, renal stone, schistosomiasis, AVM (rare), nephritic syndrome (rare). (**½ a mark for each, max 2 marks**)
2. Renal tract USS, plain KUB X-ray, flexible cystoscopy, urinary cytology. (**2**)
3. Smoking, aromatic amines (paint and dye workers), chronic cystitis, schistosomiasis (SCC), pelvic radiotherapy, cyclophosphamide. (**3**)
4. Transitional cell carcinoma. (**1**)
5. TURBT, intravesical agents (BCG or mitomycin C). (**1 mark for each, max 2 marks**)
6. Local: pelvic structures, e.g uterus, rectum, pelvic side wall.

   Lymphatic: iliac and paraaortic lymph nodes.

   Haematogenous: liver, lungs, bone. (**1 mark for each structure, max 3 marks**)

Bladder tumours are associated with smoking, male sex, aromatic amines and schistosomiasis. The majority of bladder tumours are transitional cell carcinomas (TCCs). They can present as painless haematuria, clot retention or recurrent UTIs. Investigations include urine cytology, ultrasound scanning and flexible cystoscopy. They can be diagnosed and treated at cystoscopy with transurethral resection of bladder tumour (TURBT). T2/T3 disease penetrating the muscle layer can be treated with radial cystectomy and formation of an ileal conduit where urine is passed to the anterior abdominal wall via a refashioned piece of ileum. CT scanning can assess local invasion and metastatic spread. Locally invasive and metastatic disease can be treated with palliative radiotherapy and chemotherapy. Resected tumours are followed up regularly and repeat resections are often needed.

# A³

1. Urinary tract infection, prostatitis, prostate biopsy, digital rectal examination, urinary retention, catheterisation. **(½ a mark for each, max 2 marks)**

2. Sensitivity: number of people who have the disease who test postitive (pick-up rate). OR = true positives/(true positives + false negatives).

    Positive predictive value: number of positive tests who actually have the disease. OR = true positives/(true positives + false positives). **(1 mark for each, max 2 marks)**

3. It would mean that more patients would have to undergo unnecessary secondary, possibly invasive investigations for a disease that they don't have. **(1)**

4. The course of the disease should be known, there should be an acceptable screening test for the condition, early symptoms should be present in the individual, treatment for the condition should be available to all patients, the protocol for which patients to treat should be decided, it should be a cost-effective treatment, prompt treatment should be of more benefit than delayed treatment. **(1 mark for each, max 4 marks)**

5. This is to minimise the risk of infection associated with transrectal biopsy, moving bowel flora into the prostate. **(1)**

6. Gleason score. **(1)**

7. Regular monitoring of PSA to assess if disease has progressed. **(1)**

8. Radial prostatectomy, radiotherapy/chemotherapy/brachytherapy. **(½ a mark for each, max 1 mark)**

Prostate cancer is a very common disease of elderly men. Many cases present early or are indolent in nature and require nothing more than regular surveillance. Treatment for more active disease ranges from hormonal treatment and radiotherapy to chemotherapy, minimally invasive surgery and brachytherapy. The role of PSA has been called into question for possibly causing many patients to be investigated for diseases that would not go on to kill them. Prostate biopsy is an uncomfortable experience for patients, but can be undertaken in the outpatients' department. Eventually, prostate carcinoma becomes resistant to LHRH agonists and anti-androgens. At this stage, treatment is palliative, with a median survival of 6–12 months. Other treatments are needed for complications such as bony metastases pain and chronic urinary retention. An oncological emergency may arise from spinal cord compression in patients with bone metastases.

# A4

1. Epididymo-orchitis, torted hydatid of Morgagni, testicular tumour, epididymal cyst, varicocoele, hydrocoele, inguino-scrotal hernia. **(2)**
2. Sudden-onset (usually unilateral) testicular pain, swollen and hot testis, high-lying transverse testis. **(2)**
3. Urgent scrotal exploration – scrotal ischaemia and necrosis is a time-dependent process and prompt exploration may prevent loss of testes. **(2)**
4. Skin, dartos fascia (Scarpa), external spermatic fascia, cremaster muscle, internal spermatic fascia (tunica vaginalis), tunica albuginea. **(1 mark for each, max 3 marks)**
5. To ensure that the right testis is protected from a later episode of torsion. **(1)**
6. Psychological problems associated with operation, emasculation, etc., and reduction in fertility, cosmetic deformity, reduced pubertal development if done prepuberty, and significant tissue loss. **(1 mark for each, max 2 marks)**

Acute testicular pain due to testicular torsion is a urological emergency requiring urgent surgery to preserve viable testes. It arises due to anatomical variants in the testicle with a large mesorchium which allow testicular rotation in the tunica vaginalis. Initial venous congestion evolves into arterial compression with rapid onset of testicular ischaemia and necrosis. Delays in scrotal exploration and untwisting lead to testicular death with associated atrophy. Subfertility is a serious complication of testicular torsion. Testicular torsion in young boys may be mistaken for an acute abdomen due to presence of nausea, vomiting and abdominal pain. Emergency scrotal exploration may reveal non-viable testes. In all cases, it is important to fix the contralateral testis to ensure it does not happen on that side in the future. Other causes of testicular pain include epididymo-orchitis, torsion of testicular appendages or acute inguinal lymphadenopathy.

# A⁵

1. Moves up and down with respiration, mass palpable on bimanual palpation, able to get above mass. **(2)**
2. 55 yrs old – renal cell carcinoma; 4 years old – nephroblastoma (Wilms' tumour) **(2)**
3. Varicocoele – due to compression of a renal tumour of the left renal vein, which in turn compresses the testicular vein and causes varicoele. **(2)**
4. Some renal tumours are associated with increased erythropoietin release that causes a raise in Hb. **(1)**
5. Increasing age, male gender, smoking, obesity, hypertension, long-term dialysis, hereditary papillary RCC, von Hippel-Lindau syndrome. **(½ a mark for each, max 2 marks)**
6. Stage of tumour, comorbidities including IHD, COPD, obesity. **(2)**
7. Reduced post-operative pain, reduced hospital stay, smaller incisions, reduced bleeding. **(1 mark for each, max 2 marks)**
8. Increased length of operation, poorer operative views, need for specialist equipment and training. **(1 mark for each, max 2 marks)**

Renal cell carcinoma is a malignant tumour that arises from proximal renal tubular epithelium. There is a male preponderance. Sometimes, they are asymptomatic and are found incidentally via radiological investigations for other problems. Other clinical features include haematuria, groin pain and mass in the flank. Tumours spread locally via the bloodstream after invading the renal vein and via the lymphatic system. CT scanning is useful for staging and for planning of potentially curative surgery. Extracapsular spread, renal vein and lymph node involvement confer a worse outcome. Many new techniques are available for treatment, including laparoscopic radial nephrectomy and novel monoclonal chemotherapy agents such as bevacizumab and sunitinib. These have all helped prolong survival in what can be a deadly disease.

# A⁶

1. Urinalysis. **(1)**
2. CT-KUB. **(1)**
3. The visceral nerve supply to the ureter and kidneys follows a similar course to somatic nerve supply to the gonads and flank.

Ureteric pain is then referred to these regions. Convergence in brain causes the visceral signals to be interpreted as somatic signals from the surface. **(2)**

4.  Ureteric spasm arises from peristalsis attempting to push the stone and relieve obstruction. This causes local ischaemia and hence pain. **(2)**

5.  At the renal pelvis; pelvi-ureteric junction – where the ureter passes over the pelvic brim and crosses the bifurcation of the common iliac artery; vesico-ureteric junction. **(1 mark for each, max 3 marks)**

6.  Urinary tract – infected kidney with obstruction. **(1)**

7.  Percutaneous nephrostomy to relieve infected obstruction of urine. **(1)**

8.  You do not want to insert a foreign body into a known infected space. **(1)**

9.  Increase water intake to keep hydrated. Maintain calcium intake to 1–1.2 g. Reduce oxalate-rich foods. Vitamin C reduction. **(1)**

Renal calculi are a common reason for attendance to the emergency department, and present commonly in adulthood. There may be an underlying disease, such as malignancy, hyperparathyroidism or cystinuria, that predisposes patients to forming renal stones. Most stones are calcium-based and therefore radio-opaque, and are commonly combined with oxalate or phosphate. Struvite stones form on a basis of chronic urine infection and can fill the entire calyceal system in 'stag horn' calculi. Other types of stone include uric acid, cysteine, xanthine and pyruvate. Renal colic is typically very painful intermittent stabbing pain radiating from the loin to groin, with associated microscopic or macroscopic haematuria. Infection and urine obstruction are possible complications. The mainstays of treatment are analgesia and expectant management in small stones to allow them to pass naturally. Persistent obstruction or pain mean the need for ureteric stenting and added infection may require urgent nephrostomy. Elective procedures include external shockwave lithotripsy, percutaneous or endoscopic fragmentation. Prevention centres around hydration and effective control of predisposing factors such as metabolic disorders and infection.

# A⁷

1.  Transillumination with a torch. If light transmitted, it suggests fluid-filled sac, e.g. hydrocoele. **(1)**
2.  USS testis/scrotum to assess mass and testis. **(1)**
3.  A hydrocoele arises in the tunica vaginalis. It is derived from the processus vaginalis, which is connected to the embryonic peritoneum. **(2)**
4.  Trauma, infection, tumour. **(2)**
5.  Physical: pain from increased swelling affecting walking or standing.

    Psychological: low self-esteem due to perceived differences between himself and others.

    Social: inability to take part in activities due to size, pain or embarrassment. **(1 mark for each, max 3 marks)**
6.  To ensure the fluid does not reaccumulate. **(1)**
7.  A patent processus vaginalis. **(1)**
8.  Conservative management, as most resolve spontaneously by age 1. **(1)**

Hydrocoele and scrotal swellings are a common cause of referral to urology outpatient clinics. If found under 1 year of age, most can be left alone as they are likely to resolve on their own. If they cause pain or difficulty walking, they can be operated on to allow lymphatic drainage and avoid reaccumulation. Hydrocoeles develop from a patent processus vaginalis with accumulation of fluid in the sac. On examination, they should be painless and with a penlight be able to transilluminate. Other important causes of scrotal swellings include malignant testicular lesions, traumatic haematomas, epididymo-orchitis, varicocoele, inguinal hernia or acute idiopathic scrotal oedema. Ultrasound scanning of the testis is a good way to differentiate the causes. Testicular cancer is commonly seen in young adults and is an indication for radical orchidectomy with chemoradiotherapy, depending on the stage. Tumour markers such as hCG and AFP may monitor response to treatment. Seminomas and teratomas have a good prognosis even in metastatic disease.

# A⁸

1. Bleeding, infection, atelectasis, failure of procedure, VTE, MI, risks associated with general/regional anaesthesia. **(1 mark for each, max 2 marks)**

2. Urinary continence, ability to gain an erection. **(1 mark for each, max 2 marks)**

3. Clot retention, bladder neck stenosis, bladder wall injury, retrograde ejaculation, haematospermia, TURP syndrome. **(1 mark for each, max 2 marks)**

4. Patient satisfaction, less chance of respiratory complications, quicker time to discharge, costs less, better relaxation, decreased bleeding. **(1 mark for each, max 2 marks)**

5. Irrigation fluid from the operation (glycine) enters the intravascular space via the prostatic bed and expands the intravascular space. This causes a state of fluid overload and hyponatraemia. **(2)**

Transurethral resection of the prostate is a common procedure used to treat intractable LUTS and obstructive symptoms of benign and rarely malignant prostate disease where medical therapy has failed. This can be performed under general or spinal anaesthetic. The prostate is visualised using a cystoscope and the prostate is excised using electrocautery. Irrigation with isotonic glycine keeps the operative field clear. The patient usually remains an inpatient for a short time post-operatively and an indwelling catheter is removed 24–48 hours post-operatively. Should a trial of void fail, the patient should be recatheterised and a trial of void delayed for 2 weeks. Complications include bleeding, infection, incontinence and erectile dysfunction. Newer treatments involve laser prostatectomy or microwave ablation of the prostate.

# A⁹

1. Stress incontinence: urine leaks due to raised intra-abdominal pressure as the pelvic floor and pelvic fascia fail to support the urethra so that intra-abdominal pressure + vesical pressure exceeds that of urethral closure.

   Urge incontinence: involuntary urine leak preceded by a sudden urge to micturate. This is thought to be due to overactive nerves supplying the bladder. **(1 mark for each, max 2 marks)**

2. Damage to pelvic floor during childbirth, surgery to pelvic floor, chronic cough, obesity. **(1 mark for each, max 2 marks)**

3. Weight loss, smoking cessation, avoid alcohol/caffeine/citrus/spicy food/carbonated drinks, avoid drinking at night-time, pelvic floor exercises, biofeedback, vaginal pessaries. **(½ a mark each, max 2 marks)**

4. Embarrassment to go out in public, difficulty maintaining activities as needs to be near a toilet, social stigma of incontinence. **(1)**

5. Anticholinergic. This causes less spasmodic activity. **(1)** Dry mouth, difficulty with urination, constipation, blurred vision, drowsiness and dizziness, acute closed-angle glaucoma. **(1 mark for each side effect) (max 4 marks)**

Urinary incontinence can be a distressing symptom. It is more commonly seen in women who have had children and can affect their lives adversely. It is important to define the type of incontinence, as treatment varies widely between that of urge or stress incontinence. Some forms of constant incontinence may be due to congenital abnormalities or neurological deficits. Urodynamic assessment can be used to assess different types of incontinence. Stress incontinence can be managed with pelvic floor exercises and such lifestyle changes as smoking cessation and weight loss, or surgical methods such as transvaginal tape insertion. TVT insertion may require reversal due to unacceptable urinary retention symptoms. Management of urge incontinence also focuses on such lifestyle changes as avoiding caffeine and alcohol, and bladder retraining. Other treatment for urge incontinence involves such medications as antimuscarinic or tricyclic antidepressants.

# A¹⁰

1. Bladder outflow obstruction (due to prostatic enlargement, indwelling catheter, urethral stricture), neuropathic bladder, urinary tract surgery, colovesical fistula, immunosuppression. **(1 mark for each, max 2 marks)**

2. *Escherichia coli, Staphylococcus saprophyticus, Klebsiella, Enterococcus, Proteus* sp. **(1 mark for each, max 3 marks)**

3. Pelvic trauma, perineal trauma, urethral instrumentation, urethral insertion of foreign bodies, gonorrhoea or chlamydial infections,

long-term catheter, lichen sclerosus et atrophicus. **(1 mark for each, max 2 marks)**

4. Lower urinary tract symptoms such as urgency and frequency, divergent stream, chronic retention, overflow incontinence. **(1)**

5. Urinanalysis: (MC+S and cytology), renal function (U&Es), urodynamic testing with flow cystometry and residual volume measurement, endoluminal ultrasound. **(1 mark for each, max 2 marks)**

6. Calculus formation in the urinary tract, chronic infection and spread to cause prostatitis, epididymitis or Fournier's gangrene, renal impairment due to obstruction, bladder diverticula. **(1 mark for each, max 2 marks)**

7. Bladder diverticulum is acquired because of a chronic increase in intravesical pressure causing bladder mucosa to push through the muscle layer. They can become chronically colonised with such bacteria as *Pseudomonas* or ESBL *E. coli* and cause chronic infection. **(2)**

8. Internal urethrotomy, urethroplasty, graft reconstruction, perineal urethrostomy. **(1 mark for each, max 1 mark)**

Urethral strictures occur in the background of chronic inflammation or after urethral trauma. If present in the anterior urethra, they may cause fibrosis of the corpus spongiosum, although they may affect any part of the urethra. Narrowing results from collagenous scar tissue formation in response to trauma, infection or inflammation. Lichen sclerosus et atrophicus causes dermal sclerosis and usually affects the distal urethra and urethral meatus. Symptoms include urgency, frequency, initial haematuria, incontinence or recurrent UTIs. They may be noticed incidentally when attempting urethral catheterisation for another reason. Diagnosis can be made at cystoscopy, or using radiological investigations such as uroflowmetry or voiding cystourethrogram. Many surgical interventions yield a high rate of recurrence, such as internal urethrotomy, and despite all of the treatments listed above, some patients end up requiring a suprapubic catheter.

# Trauma and orthopaedics

## A¹

1. *Staphylococcus aureus.* **(1)**
2. Blood and synovial fluid culture. **(2)**
3. ESR and CRP. **(2 marks)**
4. Analgesia **(1)**, take blood and fluid cultures (already mentioned) before empirical antibiotics. **(1)**
5. Joint washout/aspiration/debridement. **(1)**
6. *Staphylococcus epidermis.* **(1)**
7. Intra-articular injections, rheumatoid arthritis, diabetes mellitus, immunosuppression, penetrating injury, infections elsewhere, e.g. gonococcal. **(1 mark for each, max 2 marks)**

Septic arthritis should be considered in any acutely inflamed joint. Action should be prompt, as within 24 hours the joint can be completely destroyed. Some groups are susceptible to other pathogens; for example, children are more sensitive to *Haemophilus influenzae*, drug addicts to Gram-negative organisms.

## A²

1. Infraspinatus, teres minor, subscapularis. **(3)**
2. Greater tubercle. **(1)**
3. Deltoid. **(1)**
4. Teres minor, deltoid. **(2)**
5. MRI and ultrasound. **(2)**

Tears in the supraspiatus tendon are the commonest rotator cuff tear. These usually result from degeneration or less commonly from a fall or sudden jolts. The rotator cuff muscles are the supraspinatus, infraspinatus, teres minor and subscapularis. Rotator cuff tears can either be partial or complete. Complete rotator cuff tears need a prompt orthopaedic review, with a view to either open or arthroscopic repair.

# A³

1. You cannot perform a head tilt-chin lift as the cervical spine at this point is presumed unstable; therefore, you must perform jaw thrust. **(1)**
2. Nasopharyngeal tube cannot be used as there is a possibility of basal skull fracture; therefore, an oropharnygeal airway (Guedel airway). **(1)**
3. Oxygen (half mark), 15 L oxygen through a non-rebreathe mask. **(1)**
4. Insert two wide-bore cannulae, give IV fluid bolus. **(1 mark for each)**
5. FBC, U&E, cross-match, clotting (hCG in females). **(½ a mark each, max 2 marks)**
6. < 8. **(1)**
7. AP chest X-ray, AP pelvic X-ray, lateral cervical X-ray. **(1 mark for each, max 2 marks)**
8. CT head and CT abdomen. **(2)**

Any patient who has a GCS < 8 should be presumed at risk of not protecting their airway, and so a definitive airway should be sought. This means endotracheal intubation. Nasopharyngeal airways should be avoided in any patient who could have a basal skull fracture. CT scanning is a useful diagnostic tool in analysing the extent of injuries. Other methods for investigating the possibility of abdominal and pelvic trauma include a FAST scan, diagnostic peritoneal lavage, and if clinically suspicion is high enough or the patient is too unstable, then it may be necessary to take them straight to theatre for a diagnostic laparotomy.

# A⁴

1. Tension pneumothorax. **(1)**
2. Needle decompression **(1)**, a wide-bore cannula into the second intercostal space mid-clavicular line. **(1)**
3. Massive haemothorax **(1)**, wide-bore chest drain (tube thoracosotomy). **(1)**
4. Liver, heart. **(2)**
5. Chest X-ray. **(1)**
6. Chest drain. **(1)**

It is vital to check the trachea is central in every patient who presents acutely unwell. If tracheal deviation is noted with movement away from the side with breath sounds, then the cause can either be a massive haemothorax or tension pneumothorax. These conditions can lead to a patient becoming suddenly unwell. A tension pneunomothorax should be identified clinically and managed by urgent needle decompression before any imaging is organised. A massive haemothorax should be managed by draining the haemothorax. Even though a haemothorax is a 'B' (breathing) problem, a chest drain should ideally should be performed following IV access and fluids/blood given, as a large volume of fluid can be lost.

# A5

1. Anterior draw test (Lachman's test is also acceptable). **(1)**
2. Posterior draw test. **(1)**
3. Flexion of the knee to 20 degrees (loosen the cruciate ligaments and the posterior capsule), one hand then holds the ankle and the other stabilises the femur. **(1)** The knee joint is then stressed in abduction to test the medial collateral ligament and in adduction to test the lateral collateral ligament. If the knee 'opens up', it signifies that the ligament has been completely torn. **(1)**
4. Medial meniscus. **(1)**
5. Tightly adheres to the medial collateral ligament. **(1)**
6. McMurray's test. **(1)**
7. MRI. **(1)**
8. Patella tendon, hamstring tendon, quadriceps tendon. **(1 mark only)**
9. Anterior. **(1)**

Anterior cruciate ligament injuries can also follow a rotational injury at the knee where the foot remains fixed to the ground. Rest and physiotherapy can help in the management of a cruciate ligament tear, but in atheletes or if there is marked knee instability, ligament reconstruction should be considered. This is commonly from an autograft taken from the hamstrings.

# A⁶

1. Shortened, externally rotated. **(2)**
2. MRI scan, CT scan. **(1)**
3. Garden classification system. **(1)**
4. Cervical vessels in the joint capsule retinaculum, artery of the ligamentum teres, intramedullary vessels. **(2)**
5. Avascular necrosis. **(1)**
6. Arthroplasty (hemi/total). **(1)**
7. Internal fixation (nail/screws). **(1)**
8. FBC, U&Es, cross-match, clotting. **(1)**

Femoral neck fractures are a common reason for admission under orthopaedic surgeons and the incidence is rising. They are commoner in the elderly due to the increased risk of osteoporosis, osteomalacia and falls. There is often a history of trauma, but that may be trivial in patients with a predisposition to fractures. On examination, the patient will have difficulty weight-bearing and the affected leg may be shortened and rotated. Movement of the hip joint may cause pain, but patients may instead complain of knee pain with no hip pain, which is why X-rays should also be taken of the joint above and below the one affected by pain. Femoral neck fractures are subdivided into intracapsular and extracapsular fractures. Intracapsular fractures are classified by the Garden classification system. Type 1 and 2 fractures are managed by internal fixation as they are undisplaced so the blood supply to the femoral head remains intact. However, in type 3 and 4 fractures, the femoral head is removed and replaced with a prosthesis due to the disruption of the blood supply leading to the risk of avascular necrosis.

# A⁷

1. Radius. **(1)**
2. Distal metaphysis. **(1)**
3. Dorsal displacement and angulation. **(1)**
4. There is volar displacement and angulation. **(1)**
5. The arm on which the Bier's block is being performed is exsanguinated and a tourniquet is applied to the proximal part of the arm **(1)**, local anaesthetic is injected intravenously **(1)** and once the anaesthetic has taken effect the procedure to be undertaken can be performed pain-free. The tourniquet is

released after 20–30 minutes to prevent pain occurring due to the occlusion.

6. Repeat X-rays **(1)** to ensure adequate reduction. **(1)**
7. Open reduction and internal fixation, external fixation. **(1)**
8. 6–8 weeks. **(1)**

Colles' fractures are fractures of the distal metaphysis of the radius with dorsal displacement and angulation. The mechanism of action is commonly a fall on an outstretched hand in an osteoporotic patient. If there is neurovascular compromise detected on examination, urgent fracture reduction is required. Undisplaced fractures may be treated with a back-slab cast alone. Mildly displaced fractures require closed reduction, whereas fractures with severe deformity may require open reduction and internal or external fixation. A back-slab cast is then applied. A few days later, the patient is seen in fracture clinic and a full cast is applied, as the initial swelling will have subsided.

## A⁸

1. Communication between the fracture and the outside world. **(1)**
2. Gustilo and Anderson classification system. **(1)**
3. Fluid/blood resuscitation, analgesia, assessment of neurovascular status and soft tissue damage, photograph wound, sterile cover, infection and splinting, broad-spectrum antibiotics, tetanus prophylaxis, surgical debridement, surgical fracture stabilisation, wound closure. **(4)**
4. Compartment syndrome. **(1)**
5. Urgent decompression via open fasciotomy. **(1)**
6. Wound infection, tetanus infection, osteomyelitis, nerve damage, vascular damage, malunion/non-union shock, sepsis, DVT, death. **(2)**

Open fractures are classified using the Gustilo and Anderson system, which takes into account factors such as the force causing the injury, the size of the wound, the amount of soft tissue covering and the presence of vascular injury. The treatment of open fractures should be considered as an emergency. The aim is to correct shock, relieve pain, prevent infection and ensure adequate healing. Important complications to be monitored for include neurovascular damage, compartment syndrome, infection and malunion/non-union.

# A⁹

1. Conus medullaris. **(1)**
2. L2–L3. **(1)**
3. L4–L5. **(1)**
4. Fracture, haematoma, abscess, tumour, disc prolapsed. **(2)**
5. Hypotonia, hyporeflexia, weakness, muscle wasting, fasciculation. **(2)**
6. MRI scan. **(1)**
7. Urgent surgical decompression. **(1)**
8. Paralysis, sensory abnormalities, bladder dysfunction, bowel dysfunction, sexual dysfunction. **(1)**

Cauda equina syndrome is a medical emergency, and urgent investigation and management is essential to prevent complications. Clinical features include lower back pain, lower limb motor and sensory abnormalities, saddle anaesthesia and bladder and bowel dysfunction. As well as a full neurological examination of the lower limbs, a PR examination is essential to determine anal tone and sensation. MRI scans are the preferred method of investigation, but CT scans and myelography may also be used. Urgent surgical decompression is required to decrease the risk of complications occurring.

# A¹⁰

1. Females. **(1)**
2. Tenderness, derangement, swelling, decreased range of movement, pain on movement, crepitus, instability. **(2)**
3. Heberden's nodes. **(1)**
4. Joint-space narrowing, osteophytes, subchondral sclerosis, subchondral cysts. **(½ a mark each, max 2 marks)**
5. Regular exercise, weight loss. **(2)**
6. Reduced quality of life, symptoms not responding to non-surgical management. **(2)**

Osteoarthritis is the commonest condition to affect joints. The knee and hip joints are most commonly affected. Risk factors include increasing age, female sex and obesity. Pain in osteoarthritis is typically worse at the end of the day and with exercise. Rest pain occurs as the condition progresses. As well as lifestyle changes, initial management consists of analgesia, physiotherapy and walking aids. In more severe osteoarthritis, intra-articular steroid injections may provide temporary relief, but the definitive treatment is joint arthroplasty.

# ENT

## A¹

1. Trauma. **(1)**
2. Little's area/Kiesselbach's plexus. **(1)**
3. Hb may have dropped due to epistaxis; low platelets may be the cause of the epistaxis. **(2)**
4. INR as she is on warfarin, LFTs as deranged liver function may lead to insufficient synthesis of clotting factors, group and save in case transfusion is necessary. **(2)**
5. Sit patient upright and lean forwards, squeeze bottom part of the nose, apply ice pack to the bridge of the nose, monitor pulse and blood pressure, gain IV access and commence fluid resuscitation if necessary. **(2)**
6. Cauterisation, packing, balloon/foley catheter, ligation/embolisation of sphenopalatine/internal maxillary/external carotid artery. **(2)**

Epistaxis is the major ENT emergency. It is classified as anterior or posterior. Anterior epistaxis comprises the majority of cases, with bleeding often occurring from Little's area (otherwise known as Kiesselbach's plexus). This is the areas where the anterior ethmoidal, sphenopalatine and facial arteries anastamose. As with any emergency presentation, an ABCDE approach should be taken to initial management. The patient may require resuscitation with IV fluids and/or red blood cell transfusion. Obvious anterior bleeding sites may be cauterised but otherwise may require anterior packing. Posterior epistaxis may be more difficult to cauterise and can be managed by inflation of a balloon/foley catheter in addition to an anterior nasal pack. Ligation/embolisation of the arterial source is an alternative if the above measures fail to control the bleeding.

## A²

1. Odynophagia. **(1)**
2. Fever, anorexia, headache, ear pain, change in voice, abdominal pain. **(1 mark for each, max 2 marks)**
3. Jugulodigastric lymph node. **(1)**

4. Infectious mononucleosis, agranulocytosis, scarlet fever, diphtheria, malignancy. **(1 mark for each, max 2 marks)**
5. Amoxicillin will cause a maculopapular rash if the cause of the symptoms is infectious mononucleosis instead of acute tonsillitis. **(1)**
6. Analgesia, antipyretics, adequate hydration. **(2)**
7. Quinsy. **(1)**

Tonsillitis is inflammation of the tonsils caused by infection. The vast majority of infections are viral in nature, and therefore antibiotics are unlikely to be needed. The mainstay of treatment is analgesia, antipyretics and adequate hydration. Tonsillectomy is not a treatment of acute tonsillitis but aims to reduce the incidence of recurrent tonsillitis.

# A³

1. Dysphagia. **(1)**
2. This points more towards a stricture (benign or malignant) as the cause for dysphagia rather than if the difficulty was swallowing fluid as opposed to solids, when a motility disorder would be more likely. **(1)**
3. Metaplasia **(1)** of squamous to columnar epithelium **(1)** in the lower oesophagus.
4. Adenocarcinoma. **(1)**
5. Smoking, alcohol, obesity, achalasia, coeliac disease, Plummer-Vinson syndrome, increasing age, male sex, family history. **(1 mark for each, max 2 marks)**
6. TNM (Tumour, node, metastasis). **(1)**
7. Surgery, chemoradiotherapy, palliation. **(1 mark for each, max 2 marks)**

In the presence of chronic gastro-oesophageal reflux, the normal columnar epithelia of the lower oesophagus undergoes metaplasia to squamous epithelia. This process is known as Barrett's oesophagus, which leads to an increased risk of oesophageal adenocarcinoma. If localised disease is present, curative surgery may be offered or if surgery is not indicated, then chemoradiotherapy is another option. However, survival rates are poor, and often palliation is the only option.

# A⁴

1. Vagus nerve. **(1)**
2. Left, as it has a longer course than the right; therefore, it is more susceptible to damage. **(2)**
3. Cricothyroid, superior laryngeal nerve. **(2)**
4. Tumours (thyroid/oesophageal/larynx/bronchial), surgery (thyroid/parathyroid/oesophageal/cardiac), aortic arch aneurysm, bulbar/pseudobulbar palsy, idiopathic. **(1 mark for each, max 2 marks)**
5. Vocal fatigue, reduced volume of voice, shortness of breath, cough. **(1 mark for each, max 2 marks)**
6. Laryngoscopy. **(1)**

The recurrent laryngeal nerve is a branch of the vagus nerve. On the left, it extends down into the chest and courses under the arch of the aorta before ascending to the larynx. On the right, it runs under the sub-clavian artery. The recurrent laryngeal nerve supplies all the muscles of the larynx apart from the cricothyroid, which is supplied by the superior laryngeal nerve. The muscles supplied by the recurrent laryngeal nerve are responsible for the movements of the vocal cords; therefore, damage to the recurrent laryngeal nerve will cause vocal cord palsy. Unilateral vocal cord palsies can often be compensated by the other side, but bilat-eral vocal cord palsies may lead to airway occlusion, requiring urgent tracheostomy.

# A⁵

1. Strokes, cerebellopontine angle lesions, tumours, acoustic neuromas, otitis media, multiple sclerosis, Ramsay Hunt syndrome, parotid tumours, trauma, Guillain-Barré syndrome, Bell's palsy. **(½ a mark for each, max 2½ marks)**
2. Upper motor neurone lesions are 'forehead sparing'. This means that the motor innervation to the forehead is intact. This stems from the fact that the forehead is bilaterally innervated. Lesions that affect the facial nerve (lower motor lesions) will also affect the forehead. **(1)**
3. Temporal branch of the facial nerve, zygomatic branch of the facial nerve, buccal branch of the facial nerve, marginal mandibular branch of the facial nerve, cervical branch of the facial nerve. **(2½)**

4. Prednisolone – more effective if given early (within 24 hours); aciclovir – indicated if prodromal features present (ear pain, stiff neck, reddish auricle). **(2)**

5. Damage to the eye – consequence of reduced lacrimation and inability to close eye; altered taste; psychological impact. **(1 mark for each, max 2 marks)**

Bell's palsy is a lower motor neurone lesion affecting the facial nerve. It affects all the facial muscles on one half of the face – including the forehead. There is evidence that prednisolone helps if given early, within 24 hours. Bell's palsy is an idiopathic condition, and therefore is a diagnosis of exclusion, but antivirals are indicated especially in individuals where a viral cause (herpes simplex, herpes zoster (without vesicles in the auricle)) is possible. In these patients, a prodromal phase can be noted, often with pain in the ear, stiff neck or a redness noted in the auricle.

## A⁶

1. The illusion of movement: in true vertigo, the patient should be able to tell you in which direction the movement is occurring. This should be different from 'light-headedness' and 'dizziness'. **(1)**

2. Ménière's disease, vestibular neuronitis, acoustic neuroma, multiple sclerosis, cholesteatoma, trauma, drugs (gentamicin, diuretics, metronidazole, amoung others). **(½ a mark for each, max 2 marks)**

3. There is displacement of an otolith/otoconia within the semicircular canals. The heavier otolith causes abnormal movement of the endolymph within the canal, giving the sensation of vertigo. **(2)**

4. Hallpike test: if positive, the patient experiences vertigo and rotational nystagmus (after 5–10 seconds) with the fast phase towards the affected ear. After sitting up, the patient experiences more vertigo. **(1)**

5. Epley manoeuvre. **(1)**

6. Reassurance, reduce alcohol intake, medical management such as betahistine, surgical management. **(1 mark for each, max 3 marks)**

BPPV clinically manifests itself as a short-lived sensation of vertigo, often lasting around 30 seconds, typically following a turning movement of the head. It is rarely associated with deafness and tinnitus. It is associated with rotational nystagmus, with the fast phase towards the affected eye. This is due to an otolith/otoconia causing turbulence within the endolymph, resulting in the sensation of vertigo. The management and diagnosis of this condition are listed above.

# A⁷

1. Inflammation of the middle ear. **(1)**
2. *Streptococcus pneumoniae, Haemophilus influenzae, Moraxella catarrhalis.* **(2)**
3. Shorter, narrower and more horizontal – poor drainage, more likely to suffer middle ear infections. **(2)**
4. Pars flaccida, pars tensa. **(2)**
5. Bulging eardrum, reddening or dull appearance, prominent blood vessels, (+/– perforation). **(1 mark for each, max 3 marks)**
6. Antibiotics (amoxicillin) and analgesia/antipyretics. **(1 mark for each, max 2 marks)**

Otitis media often follows an upper respiratory tract infection. It often presents acutely with pain, fever and possibly vomiting and anorexia. The infection within the middle ear causes inflammation and bulging of the tympanic membrane. This pressure causes pain and can lead to a perforation of the eardrum with subsequent purulent discharge from the external acoustic meatus. Treatment is with antibiotics and symptomatic relief.

# A⁸

1. Sensorineural hearing loss in the right ear. **(1)**
2. 256–512 kHz. **(1)**
3. Mastoid process. **(1)**
4. Air conduction louder than bone conduction. **(1)**
5. Normal hearing, unilateral sensorineural hearing loss. **(1 mark for each, max 2 marks)**
6. Tuning fork placed in the midline, e.g. forehead. **(2)**
7. Benign. **(1)**
8. MRI. **(1)**
9. Meningioma. **(1)**
10. Surgery can be offered, but not all vestibuilar schwannomas need to be excised. **(1)**

Rinne's test is performed by asking the patient which is louder: a vibrating tuning fork placed on the mastoid process for bone conduction or when held in front of the ear to test air conduction. The test is said to be positive for 'normal' hearing and for sensorineural hearing loss where air conduction is louder than bone. In Weber's test, the sound should be localised to the affected ear with conductive deafness and the contralateral in sensorineural deafness. All patients presenting with unilateral sensorineural hearing loss should be investigated with MRI. The two main differential diagnoses in this case of unilateral hearing loss with tinnitus are an acoustic neuroma/vestibular schwannoma or a meningioma.

## A⁹

1. An air-filled cavity in the facial bones with connection to the nasal cavity. **(1)**
2. Maxillary, ethmoidal, sphenoid, frontal sinus. **(1 mark for each, max 4 marks)**
3. Ciliated pseudostratified columnar epithelium. **(1)**
4. Most are secondary to bacterial infection (often following a viral infection), dental root infection, diving/swimming in infected water, trauma, carcinoma. **(1 mark for each, max 2 marks)**
5. Decongestants, analgesia/antipyretics, the use of antibiotics is controversial but amoxicillin is often given. **(1 mark for each, max 2 marks)**

The paranasal sinuses can become infected by bacteria following a viral upper respiratory tract infection. This can cause mucosal oedema and so block the drainage from the sinus and also leads to impaired cilia action. This leads to stasis of mucus, which can become infected. Acutely, bed rest, decongestants and analgesia/antipyretics are advised, with antibiotic usage remaining controversial in the management.

## A¹⁰

1. Facial nerve. **(1)**
2. Submandibular, sublingual. **(1 mark for each, max 2 marks)**
3. 80%. **(1)**
4. 80% of these are pleomorphic adenomas. **(1)**
5. Pain, fast growth, fixing to other structures, facial nerve palsy. **(1 mark for each, max 2 marks)**

6. Next to the second maxillary molar tooth. **(1)**
7. Parotitis, mumps (more commonly bilaterally), duct blockage (salivary calculus). **(1 mark for each, max 2 marks)**

Around 80% of salivary gland tumours occur within the parotid gland. Around 80% of these are pleomorphic adenomas, of which 80% are in the superficial lobe. Pleomorphic adenomas usually present as a painless, mobile and slow-growing lump in middle-aged patients. These are benign lesions, but can undergo malignant transformation. They are removed by superficial parotidectomy.

# Vascular

## A1

1. An abnormal dilatation to more than 150% of original diameter of a blood vessel due to weakness in the vessel wall. **(1)**
2. A true aneurysm is an abnormal dilatation of a blood vessel, whereas a false aneurysm is a collection of blood around a blood vessel wall that communicates with the lumen. **(1)**
3. A number needed to screen is a reference to the number of patients who will need to be screened by the programme to prevent one excess death/morbidity from a ruptured AAA. **(1)**
4. AAA is a relatively rare disease. There is a significant (5%) mortality with elective surgery. **(1)**
5. Referral for surgical intervention if AAA > 5.5 cm. **(1)**
6. Atheromatous degeneration, connective tissue disorders (Ehlers–Danlos, Marfan's), mycotic aneurysms from infection. **(1 mark for each, max 2 marks)**
7. Smoking, family history, diabetes mellitus, hypertension, hyperlipidaemia, increasing age, male sex. **(½ a mark for each, max 2 marks)**
8. Bleeding, infection, DVT/PE, MI, spinal ischaemia, renal failure, mesenteric ischaemia, distal thrombus causing limb ischaemia or trash foot, death. **(½ a mark for each, max 2 marks)**
9. Multiple comorbidities making open surgery unacceptably risky; morphological aspects of AAA making it amenable to endovascular repair, position of renal arteries, tortuosity of iliac artery. **(1)**
10. Long-term follow-up is needed; it is not suitable for every type of aneurysm; high reintervention rate. **(1 mark for each, max 2 marks)**

An aneurysm is an abnormal dilatation in a blood vessel. It may occur as a result of structural abnormalities of collagen and elastin in vessel walls. Common sites for aneurysms include abdominal aorta (AAA), popliteal and iliac arteries. Atherosclerotic disease is the commonest cause of AAAs and is associated with hypertension, smoking and a family history. There is a male preponderance and they may be seen in patients with connective tissue disorders such as Marfan's syndrome or Ehlers–Danlos. True aneurysms involve all three layers of the blood vessel, whilst false aneurysms normally only contain surrounding adventitia due to trauma or arterial puncture. Diagnosis is made at rupture, incidentally or when they cause symptoms of compression of nearby structures. Recently, an AAA screening programme using abdominal ultrasound has been piloted that may reduce mortality from ruptured AAA. Elective AAAs can be repaired using endovascular stenting as opposed to an open operation.

# A²

1. Ruptured AAA. **(1)**
2. Acute pancreatitis, acute myocardial infarction, perforated abdominal viscus, renal colic/pyelonephritis. **(1 mark for each, max 2 marks)**
3. Abdominal CT scanning with IV contrast. **(1)**
4. Full blood count: Hb estimation is important, cross-match at least 6 units of red blood cells, amylase, urea and electrolytes, ECG. **(1 mark for each, max 2 marks)**
5. Red blood cells, fresh frozen plasma, platelets. **(2)**
6. Cholesterol embolism (trash foot): arises from vascular surgery where atheromatous debris is shed during surgery and travels and lodges in distal vessels, causing local ischaemia. **(2)**
7. Endothelium/intima, tunica media, tunica externa, serosa/adventitia. **(½ a mark for each, max 2 marks)**
8. Fibroblasts, macrophages, lymphocytes. **(1 mark for each, max 1 mark)**

Ruptured AAA is a life-threatening vascular emergency. The risk of rupture is directly proportional to the diameter of the aneurysm. Many patients with ruptures may not make it to hospital alive for surgical intervention. Of those that do, there is still around 50% mortality intra-operative. Once diagnosis is suspected, immediate transfer to theatre and activation of a specialist vascular surgical team give the patient the best hope of survival. Initial presentation may be of sudden collapse, upper abdominal, back and loin pain with sweating and hypotension. Immediate management includes high-flow $O_2$, establishment of large-bore bilateral IV access, urinary catheterisation, ECG and urgent cross-matching of blood. Contained leaks may initially be stable with later disastrous rupture some hours later. Surgical treatment aims to control bleeding and insert a graft. Blood products must be quickly available and post-op care is invariably on ITU. Complications include renal failure, limb ischaemia, infection and aortoenteric fistulae.

# A³

1. Acute limb ischaemia. **(1)**
2. Pallor, paraesthesia, perishing cold, paralysis. **(½ a mark for each, max 2 marks)**
3. Acute thrombosis, and emboli. Rarer causes include aortic dissection, trauma, iatrogenic injury, intra-arterial drug use and peripheral aneurysm. **(½ a mark for each, max 1 mark)**
4. Thromboembolic disease, most likely from AF. **(1)**
5. High-flow oxygen, analgesia, heparin infusion, IV fluids. **(1 mark for each, max 2 marks)**
6. Irreversible tissue ischaemia occurs within 6 hours, so limb-salvage surgery must occur before this time whilst the leg is viable. **(1)**
7. Thrombolysis, angioplasty, embolectomy, arterial bypass. **(1 mark for each, max 2 marks)**
8. Heparin activates anti-thrombin III, which in turn inactivates thrombin and factor Xa. This prevents the clotting cascade from activating fully, causing anticoagulation. **(2)**
9. Frequent monitoring of APTT and dose adjustment; increased risk of haemorrhage; heparin-induced thrombocytopenia; long-term use may cause osteoporosis. **(1 mark for each, max 2 marks)**

Acute limb ischaemia is a limb- and life-threatening emergency which requires urgent intervention to salvage limbs and prevent mortality. Ischaemia can arise from acute thrombosis in an atherosclerotic vessel or from cardiac or aneurysmal embolism. Rarer causes include aortic dissection, trauma or intra-arterial drug use. Classic clinical presentation involves pain, pallor, pulselessness, paraesthesia and perishing cold, with the last two being signs of irreversible ischaemia. Clinical assessment should elucidate the cause and viability of the limb. Immediate medical treatment includes heparin infusion, analgesia and high-flow oxygen therapy. Definitive management in salvageable limbs could involve on-table angiography, thrombolysis, angioplasty, embolectomy or arterial bypass, depending on investigation findings. In non-salvageable limbs, amputation above a level of viability is the only way to prevent fatal complications such as hyperkalaemia, acidosis and renal failure from necrotic muscle.

# A4

1. Intermittent claudication. **(1)**
2. Peripheral vascular disease – atherosclerotic disease of the peripheral circulation. **(1)** Coronary heart disease, cerebral vascular disease, mesenteric/renal artery disease, impotence, critical ischaemia, acute limb ischaemia. **(1 mark for each, max 2 marks)**
3. Smoking cessation, weight loss, diet and exercise programmes. **(1)**
4. Antihypertensives, statin therapy to improve hyperlipidaemia, antidiabetic therapy including oral therapy or insulin if required, antiplatelet agents, e.g. aspirin, clopidogrel. **(2)**
5. Critical ischaemia. **(1)**
6. This could suggest internal iliac artery stenosis, as the pudendal artery and superior gluteal arteries both arise from the iliac arteries; this could suggest proximal occlusion of the common iliac or higher, as buttock pain and impotence suggest internal iliac artery stenosis and thigh pain suggests external iliac stenosis. **(max 2 marks)**
7. Ankle brachial pressure index measurement, Doppler duplex imaging, angiogram (digital subtraction angiography), CT/MRI angiogram. **(1 mark for each, max 1 mark)**
8. U&E: renal disease can cause exacerbation of problems with IV contrast.

   Clotting: as using arterial puncture.

   Group and save: in case there is procedural blood loss.

   Glucose, lipids: assess risk factors.

   FBC: anaemia, infections, platelets.

   ESR/CRP: for possible arteritis. **(1 mark for each, max 1 mark)**

9. Common femoral artery, external iliac artery, common iliac artery, aorta. **(1)**

Intermittent claudication (from the Latin *claudicare*, to limp) is a chronic disease caused by atherosclerosis in the peripheral vasculature and is characterised by progressive burning limb pain on exertion. Diagnosis is based on clinical evaluation, and imaging such as angiography is only indicated if medical treatment has failed or surgery is planned. Medical management involves treatment of such cardiovascular risk factors as hypertension, hyperlipidaemia, diabetes and smoking. As this is a vascular disease, it may coexist with other vascular diseases, such as ischaemic heart disease or cerebral vascular disease. Surgical treatment involves angioplasty with insertion of stents or open bypass surgery of the affected segment. Bypasses include aortobifemoral and femoral-femoral crossover. Distal disease is harder to manage with bypass, with a higher rate of graft occlusion or failure. Claudication may progress to critical ischaemia, which involves rest pain and intolerance of lying leg flat. Critical ischaemia should prompt urgent surgical referral.

## A⁵

1. Transient ischaemic attack. **(1)**
2. Incidence rate is the number of new cases in a given population in a given time frame. **(1)**
3. Better control of cardiovascular risk factors; better control of AF with anticoagulation. **(1)**
4. ECG may show AF or old infarcts, both of which may cause clot formation in the heart, which can embolise to cause TIAs. **(1)**
5. Echocardiogram, carotid duplex scanning, CT/MRI head. **(1 mark for each, max 2 marks)**
6. Age, blood pressure, clinical features (weakness 2 points, speech without weakness 1 point), duration of symptoms (> 60 minutes 2 points, 10–59 minutes 1 point), diabetes present. **(2)**
7. Amaurosis fugax: caused by blocking of the central retinal artery. **(2)**
8. Death, major disabling stroke, myocardial infarction, wound haematoma. **(1 mark for each, max 2 marks)**
9. Hypoglossal nerve, ansa cervicalis, vagus nerve, internal jugular vein, superficial cervical lymph nodes. **(1 mark for each, max 2 marks)**

10. Patient is awake and can respond to commands to look for neurological deficits in real time. Avoids risks of GA. **(1)**

Carotid disease is heralded by transient ischaemic attacks (TIA) and may lead to stroke, which is a leading cause of mortality and disability in the UK. A TIA causes sudden-onset neurological deficit, which resolves within 24 hours. They occur because emboli from atherosclerotic plaques break off and lodge in the cerebral vasculature. The nature of the symptoms relates to the distribution of the artery affected and should be promptly assessed to prevent a more severe stroke. Carotid Doppler can assess carotid stenosis and surgical intervention can be offered to those with symptomatic > 70% stenosis. Carotid endarterectomy can help reduce the risk of future stroke by removing atheroma, although it carries the risk of causing a stroke in itself. Medical treatment includes antiplatelet agents and control of such cardiovascular risk factors as hypertension, smoking, cholesterol and diabetes.

# A6

1. Abnormal break in an epithelial surface. **(1)**
2. Diabetic nephropathy, diabetic retinopathy, peripheral neuropathy, increased risk of MI, stroke, peripheral vascular disease. **(½ a mark for each, max 2 marks)**
3. Venous disease, arterial disease, neuropathy, vasculitis, malignancy, infection, trauma, lymphoedema. **(½ a mark for each, max 2 marks)**
4. Neuropathic: evidence of sensory loss (in glove/stocking distribution), neuropathic deformity (claw toes, Charcot joint, loss of transverse arch, pes cavus), unrecognised repeated trauma, warm foot with bounding pulses.

   Ischaemia: cold foot, absent pulses, ulcers on toes/heel/metatarsal heads, secondary infection and surrounding cellulitis. **(3 marks)**
5. Improve diabetic glycaemic control; regular chiropody for callus removal and pressure area care; education – don't walk barefoot, wear wide-fitting shoes; treat concurrent infection; re-vascularise if indicated. **(2)**
6. Metformin can interact with IV contrast, precipitating lactic acidosis. **(1)**

7. Broad-spectrum antibiotics investigate for underlying osteomyelitis; debridement of dead tissue; drainage of pus collections; revascularisation if needed; amputation if failed medical or surgical therapy. **(1 mark for each, max 2 marks)**

8. Primary: wound edges are approximated and healing of epidermis and dermis occur without penetration and epithelialisation of the entire dermis. Produces small scars.

   Secondary: wound is open and allowed to granulate from the bottom up. Scar produced is larger and may take longer to heal. **(2)**

Diabetic foot ulcers require complex multidisciplinary care and frequently require surgery for debridement of infected tissue. Problems arise in neuropathy and lack of sensation to trivial trauma, which is then slow to heal. Treatment starts with prevention, with regular podiatry input and education to prevent minor foot trauma. Appropriate footwear with good nail care and debridement can help with prevention of foot ulcers. Risks for developing ulcers include poor diabetic control, other diabetic complications such as nephropathy and retinopathy and concurrent arterial vascular disease. In established ulceration, infection may be from atypical organisms, so broad-spectrum antimicrobials are needed. Surgery focuses on debridement, drainage of abscesses and treatment of osteomyelitis. Vascular bypasses can help if vascular disease is also present. Amputation is a considered in failed medical and surgical therapy. Inpatients require diligent care to prevent pressure ulcers and attention to hydration and glycaemic control.

# A7

1. Low molecular weight heparin, compression stockings, early mobilisation, stopping COCP 1 month prior to any major surgery, pneumatic compression intraoperative and immediately post-operative. **(1 mark for each, max 2 marks)**

2. Limb swelling and warmth, pain, erythema, mild fever, tachycardia due to inflammatory mediators, pitting oedema. **(1 mark for each, max 2 marks)**

3. Immobility, trauma, recent surgery, inherited hypercoagulability (factor V leiden, protein C/S deficiency, etc.), malignancy, smoking, polycythaemia, OCP use, dehydration, obesity, pregnancy, past DVT. **(½ a mark for each, max 2 marks)**

4. Abnormalities of the vessel wall, constituents of the blood.
   **(1 mark for each, max 2 marks)**

5. There are many reasons why a D-dimer would be high, not just DVT. For example, pregnancy, malignancy, recent surgery, inflammation. A positive test does not necessarily mean a DVT is present. **(1)**

6. Duplex USS of leg. **(1)**

7. Short-term: therapeutic dose low molecular weight heparin 1.5 mg/kg/24 hours by subcutaneous injection.

   Long-term: oral anticoagulation, e.g. warfarin to maintain INR 2–3 for 3 months for simple post-op DVT. **(1 mark for each, max 2 marks)**

8. Pulmonary embolism, venous gangrene, chronic venous insufficiency. **(1 mark for each, max 2 marks)**

9. Inferior vena cava filter: this filter is fitted via femoral/jugular vein and helps trap clots before they reach the chest. **(1)**

Venous thromboembolism is an important source of preventable mortality and morbidity in hospitals. It has been subject to intense focus from the NHS to reduce incidence by rigorous risk stratification and prophylaxis. Risk factors commonly found in hospital inpatients include immobility, trauma, recent surgery and paralysis. Pregnancy, cancer and steroid use also increase the risk. Clinical features include limb pain and swelling, erythema and oedema. Imaging with duplex ultrasound can delineate location of thrombus. Deep venous thrombosis (DVT) is very common following large surgery such as joint replacement, and USS screening is a standard post-op investigation in some centres. Pulmonary embolism (PE) is a potential complication of DVT, and presents as tachycardia, dyspnoea and pleuritic chest pain. This can be investigated with CT pulmonary angiogram. Treatment for DVT/PE is anticoagulation using oral agents such as warfarin. When commencing warfarin, it is important to give another agent such as heparin until INR is therapeutic, as warfarin is prothrombotic initially.

# A⁸

1. Major trauma, venous disease, lower limb primary malignant tumours, gas gangrene, uncontrolled sepsis or necrotising fasciitis, severely deformed limbs from neuropathic joints, failed orthopaedic surgery. **(2)**
2. Adequate blood supply to the stump to allow healing, retain as many working joints as possible, site between large joints to allow prosthesis fitting. **(2)**
3. Bones: tibia and fibula.

   Arteries: common peroneal artery, posterior tibial artery.

   Muscles: soleus, gastrocnemius, tibialis anterior, peronei longus. **(½ a mark for each, max 3 marks)**
4. Ensure correct (right) limb is marked and operated on; ensure no surrounding cellulitis at operative site. **(1)**
5. Phantom limb pain: arises from hypersensitivity of divided nerves. There is a central basis of cortical reorganisation of the primary somatosensory cortex, with proprioceptive memory meaning other stimuli cause limb pain. **(2)**
6. Antidepressants, e.g. amitriptyline; antiepileptics, e.g. gabapentin, carbamazepine. **(1)**
7. Wound infection, stump ischaemia and non-healing stump, failure to mobilise following amputation, pressure sore, arteriopathic patients may undergo cardiac events or CVAs. **(1 mark for each, max 2 marks)**
8. Haemostasis: platelets migrate to the site and a fibrin plug forms.

   Inflammation: release of inflammatory cytokines recruit macrophages and fibroblasts to the wound. A makeshift extracellular matrix forms.

   Proliferation: angiogenesis from endothelial cells and collagen production from fibroblasts occur.

   Remodelling: collagen synthesis and destruction levels out, contraction of scar takes place via myofibroblasts and surface re-epithelialises. **(½ a mark each, max 2 marks)**

Amputation is mostly performed for arterial disease, with a smaller proportion for trauma and venous disease. It is not taken lightly, and good support should be available to the patient as they are going through the process of learning to live without a limb. Amputation may be elective or emergency depending on the indication, and post-op care aims to restore mobility, function and independence. Life-threatening indications include distal gangrene, necrosis or necrotising fasciitis. The level of amputation is important, as it must allow adequate healing of viable tissue and allow the fitting of prostheses. Post-operative pain and phantom pain must be well controlled, and pain teams are important in facilitating this. Complications include infection, non-healing of wound, phantom limb pain and progression of underlying vascular disease that requires a higher level of amputation. Patients with peripheral vascular disease are at risk of perioperative cardiac events and stroke.

# A⁹

1. Valves present in superficial leg veins normally prevent retrograde flow. If these valves become incompetent, the veins dilate and become tortuous. Venous hypertension makes the valve incompetence worse and further dilatation occurs. **(2)**

2. Prolonged standing, obesity, pregnancy/COCP, family history. **(½ a mark for each, max 1 mark)**

3. External compression – gravid uterus, ovarian mass, pelvic tumour; internal obstruction – DVT; arteriovenous malformations raise venous pressure. **(2)**

4. Eczema, venous ulceration (found mostly above the medial malleolus), oedema, haemosiderin staining, lipodermatosclerosis. **(2)**

5. 5 cm below and medial to the femoral pulse. **(1)**

6. Support stockings, avoid prolonged standing, weight loss, regular walking. **(1 mark for each, max 2 marks)**

7. Bleeding, pain, ulceration, superficial phlebitis, psychological effects. **(1 mark for each, max 2 marks)**

8. Saphenous nerve: this is a branch of the femoral nerve and supplies sensory innervation to the skin on medial and anterior aspect of the calf. Damage to this nerve would produce loss of sensation and paraesthesia in this distribution. **(2)**

Varicose veins affect almost one fifth of adults and are an abnormal dilatation of leg veins due to incompetent valves that prevent the backflow of bloods. Simple treatments include compression stockings and avoiding standing for long periods. Many varicose veins are idiopathic, but secondary causes include pregnancy, pelvic masses and previous ilio-femoral DVT. Surgical treatment is usually only available on the NHS when varicose veins have a significant or adverse effect on the patient's life through bleeding, eczema, phlebitis or ulceration. Cosmetic therapies include photodynamic therapy and foam sclerotherapy. Surgical treatments include vein stripping, saphenopopliteal ligation with multiple stab avulsions and newer technologies such as laser ablation. Recurrence is a common problem with surgical interventions, and care must be taken when consenting for surgery to include possibility of bleeding and saphenous nerve damage.

## A10

1. Maintaining airway with cervical spine protection; breathing and ventilation; circulation with haemorrhage control. **(1 mark for each, max 3 marks)**
2. Direct pressure to open wound, elevation of wound, seek urgent surgical advice. **(1)**
3. Superiorly: inguinal ligament.

   Medially: medial border of adductor longus.

   Laterally: medial border of sartorius. **(1 mark for each, max. 3 marks)**
4. Femoral artery, femoral vein, femoral nerve, lymphatics. **(1 mark for each, max 2 marks)**
5. Absent or reduced distal pulses, expanding or pulsatile mass, audible thrill over mass. **(1 mark for each, max 2 marks)**
6. On table arteriogram. **(1)**
7. Gangrene, ischaemic contractures, pseudoaneurysms, amputation. **(1)**
8. Compartment syndrome: urgent fasciotomy. **(1 mark for each, max 2 marks)**

In major trauma, peripheral vascular injuries can rapidly lead to exsanguination and need prompt treatment to prevent morbidity and mortality. Blunt injury can occur from motor vehicle collisions and falls from heights. Blunt trauma is commonly associated with fractures of long bones and pelvis. In the UK, stab wounds are commoner than gunshot wounds, and along with industrial accidents account for much upper extremity trauma. Using advanced trauma life support principles, haemorrhage control and circulation maintenance is at the forefront of management and vascular injuries should be repaired in preference to major fractures. Systemic anticoagulation may be needed to ensure anastomoses and grafts remain patent after repair. Arteriography can be undertaken on table to ensure repair has been adequate. Compartment syndrome from prolonged ischaemia should be anticipated and treated with four-compartment fasciotomy to prevent muscle necrosis.

# Dermatology

## A¹

1. Symmetrical flexural. **(1)**
2. Allergic rhinitis, asthma, food allergy. **(1 mark for each, max 2 marks)**
3. Erythematous, scaly, excoriations, lichenification, crust and weeping if infected. **(1 mark for each, max 3 marks)**
4. *Staphylococcus*. **(1)**
5. Sedating antihistamines, paste bandaging, phototherapy, oral steroids, azathioprine, ciclosporin. **(1 mark for each, max 2 marks)**
6. IgE. **(1)**

Eczema is synonymous with dermatitis. It usually presents in infancy with widespread affected areas including the scalp, neck, flexor and extensor surfaces. As the child gets older, the neck, scalp and extensor surfaces are less commonly affected and the main affected areas are the flexor surfaces. Atopic eczema can sometimes have identifiable triggers, such as certain irritants, inhalants or foods. Identifying these can be an important part of management. Otherwise, management is usually with topical emollients and steroid creams; only the most severe cases require such therapy as ciclosporin or azathioprine. If the eczematous lesion becomes chronic, the skin can become lichenified, whereby there is skin thickening and exaggerated skin markings.

## A²

1. Is it itchy?
   Is it painful?
   Does it occur anywhere else?
   Has it spread?
   Does anything make it worse or better?
   Is there family history of this?
   Have you had it before, or been treated before for it?
   Any history of atopy? **(½ a mark for each, max 2 marks)**
2. Red, scaly, well demarcated. **(1 mark for each, max 2 marks)**

3. Guttate psoriasis, erythrodermic psoriasis, pustular psoriasis, flexural psoriasis. **(1 mark for each, max 2 marks)**
4. Scalp, nails, other extensor surfaces. **(1 mark for each, max 2 marks)**
5. Emollients, topical steroids, tar, vitamin D analogues (e.g. calcipotriol), vitamin A analogue (tazarotene), dithranol, phototherapy, ciclosporin, TNF-α blockers (e.g. infliximab), methotrexate. **(½ a mark for each, max 2 marks)**
6. Skin lesions which develop at a site of injury. **(1)**

Psoriasis affects approximately 2% of the population. Its commonest form is chronic plaque psoriasis; however, there are other forms of the skin disorder. It usually presents in late teens/early twenties or around the age of 60 and commonly is associated with a family history. There is hyperproliferation of the superficial skin layers, and it is this that is responsible for its red, scaly appearance. It is usually on the extensor surfaces, but can affect the flexure areas. Nail pitting and separation of nail from the nail bed (oncholysis) is an associated phenomenon. A small percentage of people with psoriasis can develop a psoriatic arthritis. It is one of the skin disorders associated with the Koebner phenomenon (as well as lichen planus and vitiligo), whereby skin lesions occur at a site of injury.

## A³

1. Pemphigus **(1)** vulgaris. **(1)**
2. Bulla. **(1)**
3. Biopsy, screen for autoantibodies. **(1 mark for each)**
4. Drug-induced; autoimmune. **(1 mark for each)**
5. Separation of skin layers (extension of blisters) when skin is rubbed. **(1)**
6. Immunosuppression/high-dose steroids. **(1)**

Pemphigus vulgaris can be a life-threatening condition that occurs most commonly in Ashkenazi Jews. It is usually mediated by an autoimmune process, whereby there are antibodies generated against the desmosomal protein which causes keratinocytes to separate from one another, causing widespread bulla formation. It can also be caused by drug reactions. Bulla usually form on the mucosal surfaces, and this is helpful in distinguishing from bullous pemphigoid (in which mucosal involvement is rare). Biopsy is usually diagnostic. Until immunosuppressive agents were readily available, pemphigus had a high mortality rate; however, even with immunosuppression it still carries a risk of death due to the disease process or side effects of the treatment.

# A4

1. Has it changed in colour, or is there variation of colour within the mole?
   Does it itch?
   Does it bleed?
   Is it symmetrical?
   Does it have an odd sensation around that area?
   Is there a family history of melanoma?
   Is it getting wider or thicker?
   Does it have a regular border? **(½ a mark for each, max 2 marks)**
2. Fair complexion, family history, sunburn, giant congenital melanocytic naevi, lentigo maligna. **(1 mark for each, max 2 marks)**
3. Lentigo maligna malignant melanoma, superficial spreading malignant melanoma, acral lentiginous malignant melanoma, nodular malignant melanoma. **(1 mark for each, max 2 marks)**
4. The (superficial to deep) thickness/Breslow thickness. **(1)**
5. Choroid of the eye, central nervous system, gastrointestinal tract. **(1 mark for each, max 2 marks)**
6. Wide local excision. **(1)**

Malignant melanomas are malignant tumours of melanocytic origin. There are four different types, of which nodular malignant melanoma is the most aggressive and carries the worst prognosis. Diagnosis of melanoma is aided by the ABCDE criteria, which helps a clinician as to when to refer a patient to the dermatologist or reassure patients; **A**symmetry of mole, **B**order irregularity, **C**olour variation, **D**iameter > 5 mm and **E**volution of the mole. Other important factors are whether it has bled, or whether it is itchy or has altered sensation. The thickness of the lesion carries the most importance in prognosis. If melanoma is metastatic, it is almost invariably fatal. Management starts with educating patients about sun exposure and the need for sun protection. Otherwise, referral to a dermatologist for excision and histological examination is required if the mole has any suspicious characteristics.

## A5

1. Squamous cell carcinoma, amelanotic melanoma, fibrous papule, sebaceous hyperplasia, actinic keratosis. **(1 mark for each, max 3 marks)**
2. Small, pearly-white nodule, telangiectasia, rolled edge, central ulcer, can be pigmented, can be cystic. **(1 mark for each, max 3 marks)**
3. Sunlight exposure/ultraviolet radiation. **(1)**
4. Mohs micrographic surgery. **(1)**
5. Reduce unnecessary sun exposure, wear sun-protection cream, wear hats and other clothing when in the sun. **(1 mark for each, max 2 marks)**

Basal cell carcinoma is the commonest skin cancer, accounting for approximately three quarters of all reported skin cancer. It most commonly occurs on the head and neck because of their exposure to sunlight. Other aetiological factors include male sex, fair skin types, immunosuppression and arsenic exposure. It is slow-growing and very rarely metastasises – it causes less than 0.01% of cancer deaths. Tumours can be categorised into low and high risk, depending on site, size and definition of margin, which can dictate treatment. Topical therapies, like imiquimod, are available or there are other options such as cryotherapy; however, surgery is usually performed to prevent recurrence. Mohs micrographic surgery involves histologically analysing samples whilst performing surgery, in order to achieve a small tumour margin and assurance that all tumour has been taken away. This gives the best cure rates.

## A6

1. Back, chest, neck. **(½ a mark for each, max 1 mark)**
2. Increased production of sebum. Pilosebaceous follicles become blocked and infected. **(2)**
3. *Propionibacterium acnes/P. acnes*. **(1)**
4. Dispel any myths that it is to do with diet or that she is unhealthy, advise that she will most likely 'grow out of it' by age 20, advise her to wash her face with soap and water twice daily. **(1 mark for each, max 1 mark)**

5.  Topical: salicylic acid, azelaic acid, benzoyl peroxide, topical antibiotics (erythromycin, clindamycin, tetracycline)

    Systemic: oral antibiotics (oxytetracycline, erythromycin, clindamycin), non-norethisterone-containing oral contraceptives (e.g. Dianette), spironolactone. **(1 mark for each answer in each category, max 2 marks)**

6.  Dry skin, dry lips, dry eyes, depression, teratogenicity, migraine, muscle aches. **(1 mark for each, max 2 marks)**

7.  To use effective contraception. **(1)**

Acne vulgaris is a common skin problem amongst teenagers due to the increase in circulating androgens causing increase in sebum production. This excess sebum production then blocks pilosebaceous follicles, which can become infected and cause an inflammatory reaction. Impacted follicles called comedones may be open or closed (also commonly known as blackheads or whiteheads). However, acne can become more than just a skin problem, with many patients also suffering with depression that can be serious enough even for patients to commit suicide, so these young patients need to be taken seriously. Patient education is required to dispel playground myths and reassure the patient. Most patients 'grow out of it', but it can progress into adulthood. The most severe cases require consultant-led isotretinoin treatment, which is highly teratogenic, and patients are often advised to use double contraception (e.g. the pill and condoms).

# A⁷

1.  Basal cell carcinoma, malignant melanoma, keratoacanthoma, pyogenic granuloma, solar keratosis, warts. **(1 mark for each, max 3 marks)**

2.  Bowen's disease. **(1)**

3.  Immunosuppression, sunlight exposure, age. **(1 mark for each, max 2 marks)**

4.  Ear, lip. **(1 mark for each)**

5.  Other skin lesions, lymphatic system. **(1 mark for each, max 1 mark)**

6.  Excision of lesion. **(1)**

Squamous cell carcinoma is the second-commonest skin cancer, accounting for approximately a fifth of skin cancers. It is a malignant tumour of the epidermal cells responsible for keratinisation, hence why the lesion oftens looks like a crusty scaly ulcer sometimes with a horny cap. Histologically, it shows disorganised keratinocytes. Other aetiological factors than previously mentioned include chronic inflammation, ionising radiation, smoking and industrial carcinogens as well the presence of solar keratoses and Bowen's disease. SCCs can be invasive and metastasise, so it is vitally important to look for evidence of spread by examining the local lymph nodes. For patients who can't tolerate surgery, radiotherapy is used instead.

## A⁸

1. Vesicles, crusting, erythematous, swollen plaques. **(1 mark for each, max 2 marks)**
2. T10. **(1)**
3. Human herpes virus 3 (HHV-3). **(1)**
4. Elderly, immunocompromised. **(1 mark for each)**
5. Analgesia, antivirals. **(1 mark for each)**
6. Post-herpetic neuralgia. **(1)**
7. Herpes zoster or human herpes virus 3 infection of the facial nerve. **(1)**

Primary infection usually occurs as chickenpox, which is experienced in childhood. After this, the virus usually lies dormant within the dorsal root ganglion. Reactivation usually occurs in old age, however immunocompromised patients can be affected at any time. The virus usually has a preeruptive phase where patients feel generally unwell and may complain of abnormal sensation or pain in the affected dermatome. After a day or two the vesicular eruption occurs, giving a classical dermatomal distribution. If the rash crosses the midline, then another diagnosis should be sought, as shingles should never cross the midline. Patients are most infective whilst the lesions are present, so patients should be educated about general hygiene and avoidance of at-risk patient groups. Antivirals only really show benefit if prescribed within 72 hours of the rash appearing.

# A⁹

1. Grade I: non-blanching erythema over intact skin.

Grade II: partial-thickness skin loss.

Grade III: full-thickness skin loss, extending into subcutaneous fat.

Grade IV: extensive destruction with involvement of muscle, bone or supporting tissue. **(1 mark for each, max 4 marks)**
2. Elderly, cardiovascular disease, obesity, poor nutrition, immobility, smoking, neurologically impaired, faecal incontinence, urinary incontinence. **(½ a mark for each, max 2 marks)**
3. Nutrition, antibiotics if infected, regular dressings, need for debridement, pain relief, patient positioning, tissue viability referral, pressure relieving mattress/chair. **(1 mark for each, max 4 marks)**

Pressure sores are a huge financial burden because of the complications they cause and the extended hospital stay that is usually associated. They are a particular problem on the elderly and stroke wards. The most useful method of tackling them is with prevention: a pressure sore assessment should be made on each patient on admission to any ward and strategies should be put in place to prevent them occurring. Strategies should include patient education, specialised mattresses and regular repositioning of mobility-impaired patients. Severe complications of pressure sores include osteomyelitis, septicaemia and death.

# A¹⁰

1. Localised scleroderma, vitiligo, squamous cell carcinoma, Bowen's disease, lichen planus, vulval intraepithelial neoplasia. **(1 mark for each, max 3 marks)**
2. Itching, dyspareunia, constipation. **(1 mark for each, max 2 marks)**
3. Biopsy, swab. **(1 mark for each, max 1 mark)**
4. Topical steroids, topical emollients, lubricants. **(1 mark for each, max 2 marks)**
5. Squamous cell carcinoma, constipation, dyspareunia, vulvodynia, uropathy, scarring. **(1 mark for each, max 2 marks)**.

Lichen sclerosus is a relatively rare skin condition, thought to be autoimmune related. The most marked symptom is itching. It commonly occurs in the perineal area in women. There is a less than 10% chance of it changing to a cancerous lesion. With this in mind, lesions are sometimes routinely biopsied. Treatment basis is topical steroids.

# Ophthalmology

## A¹

1. Infection, allergy. **(1 mark for each, max 2 marks)**
2. Trauma, acute angle-closure glaucoma, iritis, episcleritis, subconjunctival haemorrhage, scleritis. **(1 mark for each, max 3 marks)**
3. Chloramphenicol. **(1)**
4. Hygiene advice: thoroughly wash hands after using eye drops, avoid touching the eyes. **(1)**
5. *Chlamydia trachomatis*. **(1)**
6. Photophobia. **(1)**
7. Retinoblastoma. **(1)**

Conjunctivitis is a very common cause of a red eye. It is usually bilateral due to transfer of the infecting agent from one eye to the other. It is caused by infection (bacteria, usually *Staphylococcus* or viruses, usually adenovirus) or allergy. Other more serious causes must be ruled out, which is usually on history alone. As well as treating the condition, patient advice must be given to prevent spread to other family members as it is highly contagious. In the neonate, ophthalmia neonatorum is chlamydial conjunctivitis from vertical transmission at birth. This is important because it has implication for both mother and baby. Retinoblastoma must be ruled out when finding an absent red-light reflex.

## A²

1. Proliferative. **(1)**
2. Microaneurysms, flame-shaped haemorrhages, hard exudates, engorged tortuous veins. **(1 mark for each, max 3 marks)**
3. Ishcaemic nerve fibres. **(1)**
4. Panretinal photocoagulation. **(1)**
5. Maculopathy. **(1)**
6. Cataract, glaucoma, vitreous haemorrhage, retinal detachment, ocular motor nerve palsies, infection. **(1 mark for each, max 2 marks)**
7. Good glycaemic control. **(1)**

Diabetic eye disease is most commonly manifested as diabetic retinopathy. There are characteristic changes associated with this. It travels through the stages of background retinopathy denoted as presence of microaneurysms. Preproliferative retinopathy is denoted by cotton wool spots and flame-shaped haemorrhages, which mark the presence of ischaemia at the retina. Finally, proliferative retinopathy is denoted by the presence of new vessels at or around the optic disc. Maculopathy can also be present. Treatment for diabetic retinopathy is by panretinal photocoagulation with the aim of causing a regression in the new blood vessels. Diabetics are at high risk of many other eye conditions, and good glycaemic control is the aim for prevention of these occurring.

## A³

1. Graded 1–4. **(1)**
2. Arteriolar constriction (silver/copper wiring), arteries nipping veins where they cross (AV nipping), cotton wool spots or exudates, flame-shaped haemorrhages, papillloedema. **(1 mark for each, max 4 marks)**
3. Arteriolar constriction and arteries nipping veins where they cross (silver/copper wiring and AV nipping). **(2)**
4. Calcium channel blocker. **(1)**
5. Papilloedema. **(1)**
6. Phaeochromocytoma. **(1)**

Hypertensive retinopathy is usually asymptomatic; it is associated with a chronic elevation in blood pressure. The severe end of the spectrum at grade 4 involving papilloedema is only usually associated with malignant hypertension, and an underlying disorder must be searched for. Patients with hypertensive retinopathy are at risk of retinal vein or retinal artery occlusion. The mainstay of treatment of hypertensive retinopathy is with good blood pressure control. Calcium channel blockers are first-line agents for patients over the age of 55 years, with thiazide diuretics as second-line. In the under-55 age group (not of African origin), ACE inhibitors are first-line.

## A⁴

1. Do you have any pain in the eye(s)?
   Is the visual loss central or peripheral?
   Is the visual loss sudden or gradual?

Is it bilateral or unilateral?

Is it associated with a red eye?

Any symptoms of stroke, such as weakness on one side?

Has there been any trauma?

Was it like a curtain descending?

Any headache associated?

Does it hurt to move your eyes? (½ a mark for each, max 3 marks)

2. Maculopathy, retinal disease, presbyopia, optic neuritis, vitreous haemorrhage, giant cell arteritis, transient ischaemic attack, retinal vein occlusion, central retinal artery occlusion, optic atrophy, macular degeneration. (½ a mark for each, max 1 mark)

3. Diabetes, eye trauma, uveitis, long-term steroids, smoking, congenital, myotonic dystrophy, radiotherapy/radiation. (1 mark for each, max 2 marks)

4. Clouding of the lens, absent red-light reflex. (1 mark for each)

5. Phacoemulsification. (1)

6. Early – posterior capsule rupture; late – posterior capsule opacification. (1 mark for each)

A cataract is an opacity of the lens. Cataracts are the leading cause of blindness in the world. In the UK, they are more associated with the elderly population; however, cataracts can be congenital usually due to maternal infection, e.g. rubella. Patients with developing cataract usually complain of gradual visual disturbances, such as having trouble reading the paper or not recognising faces. Other symptoms are seeing 'haloes' when the sun is in their eyes. Phacoemulsification involves breaking up the affected lens with ultrasound then aspirating it through a cannula. A replacement artificial lens is then inserted. The posterior capsule is left 'untouched' at surgery to make surgery safer; however, it is the source of the commonest complication; opacification, which is treated with laser therapy.

## A5

1. Tonometer; 21. (1 mark for each)

2. Gonioscopy is the measurement of the iridocorneal angle. It is important to distinguish between open- and closed-angle glaucoma. (2)

3. Optic disc and evidence of optic disc cupping. (1)

4. Age, family history, race, myopia, intraocular hypertension.
   **(1 mark for each, max 2 marks)**
5. Prostaglandin analogues, β-blockers, carbonic anyhdrase inhibitors, miotics, sympthomimetic agents. **(½ a mark for each, max 2 marks)**
6. DVLA. **(1)**

Open-angle glaucoma, also known as chronic simple glaucoma, is usually asymptomatic until visual field defects occur. It is characterised by optic neuropathy and usually occurs in the presence of intraocular hypertension, but not always. Family history and race are strong risk factors – there is higher incidence in Afro-Caribbeans. The most marked risk factor for glaucoma is raised intraocular pressure. Elevated intraocular pressure causes nerve compression and death (this is seen as 'optic disc' cupping), normal cup : disc ratio is < 0.5, but in glaucoma it can be as high as 0.9–1.0. Patients with glaucoma need screening annually for intraocular pressure measurement and assessment of their optic disc. Treatment cannot reverse any optic nerve damage, but can prevent progression.

## A6

1. Wet. **(1)**
2. Amsler chart, slit-lamp fundoscopy, optical coherence tomography (OCT), fluorescein angiography. **(1 mark for each, max 2 marks)**
3. Drusen, atrophic change, choroidal neovascularisation (CNV), leaking blood vessels. **(1 mark for each, max 2 marks)**
4. Photodynamic therapy (with use of verteporfin), laser photocoagulation, intravitreal vascular endothelial growth inhibitors (anti-VEGF). **(1 mark for each, max 3 marks)**
5. Advise to inform DVLA, stop smoking, eat diet rich in green vegetables, inform patient it will not cause complete blindness and should only affect central vision. **(1 mark for each, max 2 marks)**

ARMD is the commonest cause of blindness in the UK. It occurs in the elderly and affects central vision. It is characterised by deposition of drusen, which is the deposition of abnormal hyaline material between the retinal pigment epithelium and Bruch's membrane of the retina. Also, when looking at the retina the macula can have a pale mottled appearance which correlates to atrophy of the retina. The most notifiable risk factors are increasing age and smoking. It has two forms 'wet' and 'dry'.

The dry type is associated solely with the changes mentioned above and is slowly progressive; however, the wet type is associated with a more rapid decline in vision due to the development of new leaky vessels growing from the choroid into the neurosensory retina – this is called choroidal neovascularisation. These new vessels push the retina forwards, which gives the symptoms of distorted vision, particularly of wavy lines as mentioned in the clinical case. This is tested for using an Amsler chart. Optical coherence tomography gives a cross-section of the retina which can help visualise changes at the retina.

## A7

1. Family history, female gender, hypermetropia, increasing age.
   **(1 mark for each, max 1 mark)**
2. Decreased visual acuity, hazy cornea, large fixed dilated pupil, increased intraocular pressure, circumcorneal injection (redness).
   **(1 mark for each, max 4 marks)**
3. Corneal oedema. **(1)**
4. Pupil constricts on going to sleep and so pulls the peripheral iris out of the angle. **(1)**
5. Acetazolamide, pilocarpine, mannitol, topical steroids, topical β-blocker, prostaglandin analogue, alpha-adrenergic analogue.
   **(1 mark for each, max 2 marks)**
6. Peripheral iridectomy. **(1)**

AACG usually occurs after the age of 40 and is one of the top differentials for an acutely painful red eye. It occurs when the drainage of aqueous fluid becomes blocked due to the iris being pushed up against the trabecular meshwork; this then increases intraocular pressure. The rapid increase in pressure causes the cornea to become oedematous, which causes blurring of vision, and the pupil can become fixed due to the iris sphincter becoming ischaemic. People who are long-sighted are at particular risk due to the anterior chamber being shallow and having a small angle. The condition particularly occurs at night, when the pupil is more dilated and the iris bunches up in the corner, which causes angle closure. After reducing intraocular pressure medically and constricting the pupil to hopefully open the angle, treatment is ultimately with peripheral iridectomy to allow free movement of aqueous. This is done in both eyes to reduce the risk of recurrence in either eye.

# A⁸

1. Optic neuropathy, vitreous haemorrhage, central retinal artery occlusion, retinal vein occlusion, cerebrovascular accident. **(1 mark for each, max 3 marks)**
2. Lower half of retina. **(1)**
3. Floaters, flashes, decreased visual acuity. **(1 mark for each, max 2 marks)**
4. Myopia, due to thinning of retina as it is stretched over a larger area. **(2)**
5. Cryotherapy, laser therapy, vitrectomy, scleral buckle, pneumatic retinopexy. **(1 mark for each, max 2 marks)**

Sudden painless loss of vision has a host of causes, as mentioned above. With retinal detachment, the diagnosis usually comes from history-taking. It involves the sensory retina detaching from the retinal pigmented epithelium beneath. Retinal detachment can be classified into two groups – rhegmatogenous and non-rhegmatogenous. Rhegmatogenous retinal detachment occurs due to a break or tear in the sensory retina, whereas non-rhegmatogenous retinal detachment occurs where the sensory retina is either pulled off (tractional) or pushed off (exudative) the retinal pigmented epithelium. The location of retinal detachment can be identified from the area of visual loss, i.e. if the visual loss is superior, the detachment has occurred on the inferior aspect of the retina and vice versa. On fundoscopy, the area of detachment appears as a sheet of sensory retina ballooning forward; a tear may also be visualised. Treatment for large retinal detachments is always surgery, with the aim of opposing the two separated layers. Small tears in the retina which may cause detachment can more appropriately be treated with laser or cryotherapy.

# A⁹

1. Acuity, pupillary responses, eye movement, fundoscopy, corneal sensation, visual fields, the external eye. **(½ a mark for each, max 2 marks)**
2. Blood pressure, auscultate the carotids for possible bruits, auscultate the heart for possible murmurs, feel pulse for possible atrial fibrillation. **(1 mark for each, max 2 marks)**
3. Thromboembolism. **(1)**
4. Giant cell arteritis/temporal arteritis. **(1)**

5. An afferent pupillary defect of the right eye. **(1)**
6. Pale retina, cherry-red spot at the macula. **(1)**
7. Intravenous steroids/high-dose steroids. **(1)**
8. Yes. **(1)**

Central retinal artery occlusion is one of the differential diagnoses of sudden painless loss of vision. With this particular clinical problem, a general examination should be performed as well as taking a good past medical history in order to find a root cause. The commonest cause is a thromboembolic event, hence the need for a brief cardiovascular examination. On examination of the eyes, the afferent pupillary defect will be the first noticeable sign (this is seen as an absence of pupillary constriction when a light is shone into the affected eye, whilst there will be pupillary constriction in the affected eye if light is shone into the non-affected eye). The retina will appear pale due to ischaemia, but a cherry-red spot will be evident at the macula due to blood supply coming from the underlying choroid. If central retinal vein occlusion is due to an inflammatory process, such as temporal arteritis (as in the clinical case described), then high-dose steroids are required as soon as possible, as there is only a 6-hour window in which to save the patient's sight.

# A¹⁰

1. Human herpes virus 3 (HHV-3). **(1)**
2. Burning, itching, paresthesia, headache, fever, myalgia. **(½ mark for each, max 1 mark)**
3. Dermatomal. **(1)**
4. Nasociliary nerve; means there will be likely corneal involvement, with a loss of corneal sensation leaving the cornea vulnerable to abrasion; Hutchinson's sign. **(1 mark for each)**
5. Fluorescein. **(1)**
6. Dendritic. **(1)**
7. Corneal sensation; this may be affected in ophthalmic shingles and can leave the eye exposed to corneal ulceration. **(1 mark for each)**

Shingles is a human herpes virus which usually lies dormant in the dorsal root ganglion, or in the case of ophthalmic shingles, the trigeminal nerve root ganglion. This dormant episode follows primary infection as a child with chickenpox. Ophthalmic shingles usually occurs in the elderly population. Approximately 50% of cases of ophthalmic shingles will have nasociliary nerve involvement (Hutchinson's sign). This is a bad prognostic sign, as it means the possibility of eye involvement. On examination, the patient will have an absence of the blink reflex when the cornea is touched lightly with some cotton wool. This then leaves the cornea exposed to abrasion. Examination of the cornea with blue light and fluorescein is needed to look for the characteristic dendritic ulcers associated with ophthalmic shingles. Management of ophthalmic shingles is specialist-led and may involve antivirals, topical steroids or topical antibiotics.

# Obstetrics

1. Twin/multiple pregnancy, in women of high parity, older pregnant women, scarred uterus (previous Caesarean section). **(1 mark for each, max 2 marks)**
2. Bleeding from the genital tract after 24 weeks' gestation. **(1)**
3. Placental abruption; incidental genital tract pathology, e.g. cervical cancer, cervical polyp; uterine rupture; vasa praevia. **(1 mark for each, max 2 marks)**
4. Can provoke massive bleeding. **(1)**
5. Ultrasound scan, full blood count, clotting studies, group and save/cross-match, cardiotocography. **(1 mark for each, max 3 marks)**
6. Anti-D. **(1)**

Antepartum haemorrhage is bleeding from the genital tract after 24 weeks' gestation. This is the time at which neonatal survival is better. Placenta praevia occurs when the placenta implants in the lower segment of the uterus. It complicates about one in 200 pregnancies at term. It can be classified as 'marginal' (placenta in lower uterine segment not covering the os) or 'major' (placenta partially or completely covering the os). If the placenta is in the lower segment, it can obstruct engagement of the foetal head, leaving it lying high and not engaged, and commonly the lie may be tranverse or breech; this can be felt on examination. It may necessitate Caesarean section. Haemorrhage can be large. Post-partum haemorrhage can be severe because the lower uterine segment is unable to contract down and shear off the maternal blood supply. Anti-D is given to rhesus-negative women, and steroids are administered if gestation is less than 34 weeks. If Caesarean section is required, it is usually done electively at 39 weeks. If blood loss is severe at presentation, an emergency Caesarean section may need to be performed, but usually the patient can be monitored and transfused with blood products until 39 weeks.

# A²

1. Abdominal pain. **(1)**
2. Separation of (part or all) the placenta prior to delivery. **(1)**
3. Normal (longitudinal lie and cephalic presentation). **(1)**
4. Intrauterine growth restriction, previous abruption, maternal smoking, pre-eclampsia, hypertension, multiple pregnancy. **(½ a mark for each, max 1 mark)**
5. Degree of shock is out of keeping with visual loss. This is due to the blood not escaping from the uterus; this is 'concealed' loss because the bleed is retroplacental. **(2)**
6. Caesarean section. **(1)**
7. Afibrinogenaemia: this is due to placental damage causing release of thromboplastin into the circulation, which leads to disseminated intravascular coagulation and afibrinogenaemia due to clotting factors and in particular fibrinogen being 'used up'. **(2)**
8. Foetal blood vessels running in front of presenting part. **(1)**

Placental abruption has important contrasts with placenta praevia, as in the table below. It can be classified as 'revealed' or 'concealed'. Revealed is when the major haemorrhage is apparent externally; concealed is when the majority of the bleeding is contained between the placenta and uterine wall. With concealed abruption, the patient will often be in labour and the foetal sounds may be absent in up to a third of cases. Vasa praevia is a rare condition. If the vessel running in front of the presenting part ruptures, it can lead to massive blood loss and foetal loss is very high. The presentation is painless vaginal bleeding accompanied by severe foetal distress.

| Placenta Praevia | Placental Abruption |
|---|---|
| Shock in proportion to visual loss | Shock not proportional to visual loss |
| Pain absent | Pain usually constant with exacerbations |
| Uterus non-tender | Tense, tender uterus |
| Lie/presentation may be abnormal | Lie/presentation usually normal |
| Foetal heart sounds normal | Foetal heart sounds distressed or absent |
| Coagulation problems are rare | Coagulation problems can occur |
| Blood usually bright red fresh blood | Blood can be darkened 'old blood' |

# A³

1. Human chorionic gonadotrophin (hCG). **(1)**
2. 12 weeks. **(1)**
3. 21 November. **(1)**
4. Haemoglobin or full blood count, blood group and rhesus status, rubella, immunity, syphilis serology, blood glucose levels, HIV, hepatitis B; haemoglobin electrophoresis to test for sickle-cell disease. **(½ a mark for each, max 2 marks)**
5. Screening for sexual infection, eg. chlamydia; risk of premature delivery; vertical transmission, e.g. neonatal conjunctivits. **(1 mark for each, max 2 marks)**
6. Cardiac abnormalities, other structural abnormalities. **(1)**
7. Alpha fetaprotein decreased, unconjugated oestriol decreased, human chorionic gonadotrophin increased. **(1 mark for each, max 2 marks)**

The commonest cause of secondary amenorrhoea is pregnancy and secondary omenorrhoea is the commonest reason why pregnancy is suspected. Pregnancy is routinely confirmed on urine testing but can also be confirmed from a blood test, which will give a postive test earlier in the gestation than that of urine testing. Naegele's rule is used for estimating the due date:

First day of last menstrual period – 3 months + 7 days + 1 year

A range of blood tests is offered on the booking visit at usually 9–11 weeks' gestation. An ultrasound scan is offered to confirm gestation and viability and will diagnose multiple pregnancy if present. It can also be used for screening for chromosomal abnormality, i.e. nuchal translucency. The triple test can be used in conjunction with nuchal translucency and the blood test is usually done between 15 and 20 weeks' gestation.

# A⁴

1. Previous history of gestional diabetes; previous foetus > 4 kg; previous unexplained stillbirth; first-degree relative with diabetes; BMI> 30; family origin with high prevalence of diabetes, e.g. Asian, black Caribbean. **(1 mark for each, max 3 marks)**

2. An increase in foetal blood glucose brings about a hyperinsulinaemia in the foetus, leading to increased fat deposition. **(2)**

3. Congenital abnormalities, preterm labour, foetal lung maturity at any gestation is less than non-diabetic pregnancies, increased birth weight, polyhydramnios, shoulder dystocia/birth trauma, sudden foetal death. **(1 mark for each, max 2 marks)**

4. Hypoglycaemia. **(1)**

5. She is at a higher risk of developing diabetes in the future; she is also at a higher risk of developing gestational diabetes in future pregnancies. **(1 mark for each)**

Gestational diabetes is the development of glucose intolerance in pregnancy that disappears at the end of pregnancy. Pregnancy is 'diabetogenic'. The urinary threshold of glucose in the non-pregnant kidney is approximately 11 mmol/L, but this falls in pregnancy so much that it may reach threshold at relatively normal blood glucose levels. Foetal complications of this are as described in the answers. Insulin requirements usually increase and hypoglycaemia may result as a result of attempts to achieve optimum glucose control. Preconceptual care for the diabetic woman planning a pregnancy should have glucose control optimised and start folic acid at high dose. Close monitoring during pregnancy is required, and visits are usually alternate weeks and weekly after 34 weeks. Insulin is the mainstay of treatment; oral agents are seldom used. A special cardiac scan is required as well as serial growth scans. Elective Caesarean is often advised if the foetal weight is above 4 kg. The neonate commonly develops hypoglycaemia as a result of hyperinsulinaemia because it has been 'used to' high circulating glucose levels.

## A5

1. Post-partum (puerperal) psychosis. **(1)**

2. Nearly always within the first 2 weeks. Usually 3–5 days. **(1)**

3. There is an increased risk of her developing mental illness in later life and there is approximately a 50% chance of post-partum psychosis recurring after future pregnancies. **(2)**

4. In the first 3 months. **(1)**

5. 5%–15% **(1)**

6. Previous post-partum depression, previous depression or bipolar disorder, lack of social support, marital/partner relationship problems, recent stressful life events. **(1 mark for each, max 2 marks)**

7. Post-partum thyroiditis. **(1)**

8. Change in hormone levels. **(1)**

Psychiatric issues are common after pregnancy. The most striking of all is post-partum psychosis which occurs in approximately 0.2% of women. Onset is abrupt and early after delivery, usually in 48 or 72 hours. The recurrence of this is high, at approximately 50% in subsequent pregnancies. Treatment usually requires specialist mother-and-baby units, tranquilising medication and involvement of a psychiatrist. Post-partum depression is commoner, with approximately 5% of pregnant women suffering; however, the actual figure is believed to be closer to 10% because of women who do not present to healthcare services with the problem. Future mental health issues are closely associated. The 'baby blues' are believed to be caused by a change in the hormonal state as well as psychosocial issues. They occur in reportedly up to 50% of women. Onset is usually within the first few weeks and responds well to emotional support, usually resolving within a day or so.

## A6

1. Blood pressures of greater than 140/90 and presence of proteinurea (> 0.3 g/24 h) after 20 weeks of pregnancy. **(1)**

2. Nulliparity, multiple gestation, previous history, family history, diabetes, pre-existing hypertension, older maternal age, obesity, antiphospolipid syndrome and other autoimmune disease. **(½ a mark for each, max 3 marks)**

3. Headache, visual disturbance, nausea and vomiting, epigastric pain, brisk reflexes, clonus, acute oedema. **(½ a mark for each, max 2 marks)**

4. Labetalol, nifedipine, hydralazine, methyldopa. **(1 mark for each, max 2 marks)**

5. Magnesium sulphate, checking reflexes. **(1 mark for each)**

6. Haemolysis, elevated liver enzymes (ALT and AST), low platelets. **(1)**

Pre-eclampsia is an important obstetric topic and a significant cause of direct maternal obstetric death. Patients usually present via a community midwife after a home visit. Patients are usually asymptomatic. The pathophysiology is not completely understood; however, there is incomplete trophoblastic invasion of spiral arterioles in the placental bed. This can eventually cause diffuse endothelial damage in the mother and lead to hypertension, but with other complications such as pulmonary oedema, renal failure and cerebrovascular haemorrhage on the severe end of the spectrum. In the foetus, this leads to intrauterine growth restriction. Pre-eclampsia is also associated with placental abruption. Treatment is with antihypertensive agents in the early stages. Magnesium sulphate is used if the clinician believes eclampsia (a seizure secondary to pre-eclampsia) is imminent or has occurred. It needs close monitoring as it is associated with decreased consciousness, respiratory depression and profound hypotension, but diminishing of the reflexes is the first sign of toxicity. HELLP syndrome is linked to pre-eclampsia, and this is the reason for doing an FBC, LFT, urate levels and U&Es on patients presenting with pre-eclampsia. HELLP syndrome is also the cause for the epigastric pain which is sometimes the presenting symptom.

## A⁷

1. Preterm prelabour rupture of membranes. **(1)**
2. Erythromycin. **(1)** Steroids: betamethasone/dexamethasone. **(1)**
3. Maternal: pyrexia, tachycardia, hypotension, offensive discharge, uterine tenderness. **(1)**

   Foetal: tachycardia. **(1)**
4. Induction of labour. **(1)**
5. Cervical dilatation, station of foetal head, position of cervix, effacement of cervix, consistency of cervix. **(1 mark for each, max 5 marks)**
6. Vaginal prostaglandins. **(1)**

The recommended management for preterm prelabour rupture of membranes is with erythromycin and steroids. Tocolytics such as tractocile have shown no clinical benefit in terms of foetal outcome and so are not routinely used. The Oracle trial also highlighted that the use of erythromycin is the preferred choice of antibiotic to prevent infection compared to co-amoxiclav, as this was associated with an increase incidence of necrotising enterocolitis in the neonatal period. When a patient ruptures membranes at term (> 37 weeks), the majority will go into labour within 24 hours; if not, then induction of labour is required. A Bishop score is calculated from the five components; each component can score up to 2 or 3 depending on examination findings. A score of 5 or more is favourable for induction of labour.

# A⁸

1. On history: painful calf, cough, haemoptysis, pleuritic chest pain.

   On examination: cyanosis, tachycardia, pleural rub, decreased breath sounds, raised JVP. (**½ a mark for each, max 2 marks**)
2. Start low molecular weight heparin at therapeutic dose. **(1)**
3. Computed tomographic pulmonary angiogram (CTPA) or ventilation perfusion scan (V/Q). **(1)**
4. Underlying antiphospholipid syndrome. **(1)**
5. Previous deep vein thrombosis or pulmonary embolism, family history, malignancy, obesity, pregnancy, thrombophilia, severe infection, immobility, recent surgery, combined oral contraceptive pill use. (**1 mark for each, max 3 marks**)
6. The gravid uterus puts greater pressure on the left iliac vein at the point it crosses the left iliac artery, slowing venous return to the heart. **(1)**

Venous thromboembolism (VTE) is the foremost direct cause of death amongst pregnant women! It's a diagnosis that should never be missed and there should be a low threshold of suspicion. This lady is likely to be suffering from antiphospholipid syndrome in light of her previous history. Antiphospholipid syndrome is routinely screened for if a patient has recurrent miscarriages (three or more). It is also a cause for pre-eclampsia in pregnancies that continue beyond 20 weeks. There are many risk factors for VTE, but pregnancy is a significant one. A women is at least 10 times the risk of suffering VTE when pregnant. This is due to an increase in clotting factors, a change in the blood flow due to mechanical obstruction and less fibrinolysis. A deep vein thrombosis is nine times more likely to occur in the left leg than the right. It is important to also remember that a CTPA or V/Q scan is not contraindicated in pregnancy, despite foetal exposure to radiation.

# A⁹

1. $G_5P_2$. **(1)**
2. Bile acids, liver function tests. **(1 mark for each)**
3. Previous stillbirth. **(1)**
4. Premature delivery (spontaneous or iatrogenic); stillbirth; sleep deprivation of mother. **(1 mark for each, max 2 marks)**
5. Ursodeoxycholic acid, antihistamines, topical emollients. **(1 mark for each, max 2 marks)**
6. Induction of labour. **(1)**
7. There is an increased risk of recurrence compared to the general population. **(1)**

Obstretic cholestasis is a diagnosis of exclusion. Once other causes for deranged liver functions tests are ruled out and causes for pruritis are ruled out, then a diagnosis of obstetric cholestasis can be made. Other blood tests that may be used are viral screens, autoimmune screens, cytomegalovirus or Epstein-Barr virus blood tests. It always resolves after delivery. The risks of obstetric cholestasis are listed in the answers. This is why patients with the diagnosis are managed in a consultant-led clinic and often early induction of labour is discussed and offered.

# A¹⁰

1. Prelabour: previous shoulder dystocia, high maternal body mass index, large foetus, diabetes

   Intrapartum: prolonged first stage of labour, prolonged second stage of labour, oxytocin augmentation, secondary arrest. **(1 mark for each, max 2 marks)**
2. McRoberts manoeuvre – hyperflexion of the maternal hips (knees up to the chest). **(1)**

   Suprapubic pressure. **(1)**
3. A – appearance (skin colour)
   P – pulse rate
   G – grimace (reflex irritability)
   A – activity (muscle tone)
   R – respiration (breathing). **(1 mark for each, max 5 marks)**

4. The list is long. These are the commonest causes: polyhydramnios, prematurity, abnormal lie (transverse, oblique), foetal abnormalities, abnormal placentation, artificial rupture of membranes, breech presentation, unengaged presenting part. (½ a mark for each, max 2 marks)

5. Taking pressure off the cord by lifting the baby's head. (1)

6. Emergency Caesarean section. (1)

Shoulder dystocia and cord prolapse are two obstetric emergencies. Management of both of these emergencies should start prior to the time they present. Risk factors for both should be identified antenatally and managed accordingly, for example, a mother with a baby in breech presentation should be offered an elective Caesarean section as well as a mother who is diabetic with a grossly macrosomic foetus. Other manoevres used in management of shoulder dystocia include internal rotation, delivery of posterior arm, bending or breaking of foetal clavicle, division of the symphysis pubis; however, greater than 90% of shoulder dystocia cases are resolved with the McRoberts and suprapubic pressure. A mother who is not fully dilated with a cord prolapse will need immediate Caesarean section; however, if fully dilated then normal delivery should be expedited as soon as possible.

## A¹¹

1. Yes. Due to physiological anaemia. (2)
2. No. Due to hyperdynamic circulation. (2)
3. Increase their tidal volume. (1)
4. Foetal heart rate 110–160 beats per minute, presence of accelerations, variability of greater than 5 beats per minute, absence of decelerations. (2)
5. Maternal infection, foetal bleeding disorder, prematurity, abnormal presentation. (1 mark for each, max 2 marks)
6. 7.25 (1)

Physiology changes quite dramatically during pregnancy. A physiological anaemia occurs due to an increase in plasma volume by 1 L and only an increase of red cell mass of 300 mls, therefore causing a haemodilution. Cardiac output increases by around 40%, heart rate increases and there is also an increase in stroke volume. This creates a hyperdynamic circulation, and an ejection systolic murmur is heard in up to 90% of pregnant women. It is often thought that women's respiratory rate increases to compensate for the increase in oxygen demand; however, this is not true, and in fact they increase their tidal volume and therefore reduce their residual volume. Foetal blood sampling is a useful tool when there is a suspicious CTG trace. A borderline value of 7.20–7.24 usually indicates a repeat sample after 30 minutes to an hour, while a sample of below 7.20 indicates immediate Caesarean section.

# Gynaecology

A¹

1. Acute appendicitis, ovarian cyst disease, renal colic. **(1 mark for each, max 2 marks)**
2. Amenorrhoea, vaginal bleeding, tachycardia, hypotension, shoulder tip pain, cervical excitation, adnexal mass. **(1 mark for each, max 2 marks)**
3. Urine βhCG. **(1)**
4. Transabdominal and transvaginal ultrasound scanning. **(1)**
5. Previous pelvic inflammatory diease (e.g. chlamydia), previous tubal surgery, previous ectopic pregnancy, endometriosis, progesterone-only pill, presence of intrauterine contraceptive device, previous sterilisation. **(1 mark for each, max 2 marks)**
6. Fallopian tube, ovary, cervix, peritoneum, liver. **(1 mark for each, max 2 marks)**
7. Laparotomy/laparoscopy with salpingectomy or salpingostomy. **(1)**
8. IM methotrexate **(1)**
9. Injection of anti-D immunoglobulin. **(1)**

Ectopic pregnancy is the situation where the fertilised ovum implants in a site outside of the uterine cavity. Ectopic pregnancy is the leading cause of maternal mortality in the first trimester. Most ectopic pregnancies implant in the Fallopian tubes, although other sites include ovary, cervix and peritoneum. Risk factors include salpingitis, past ectopic pregnancy, endometriosis and older IUCDs. Presentation may be from rupture, which causes sudden severe pain, bleeding and peritonism, and can lead to haemodynamic instability. Patients may present before rupture with dark PV bleeding and tubal colic. If the patient is blood-group-negative, administration of anti-D is important. Unstable patients require urgent laparotomy and control of intraperitoneal haemorrhage. Laparoscopy can be performed if diagnosis is made and the patient is stable. Small ectopics with a low βhCG can be managed with methotrexate or expectantly.

# A²

1. Hyperemesis gravidarum. **(1)**
2. First pregnancy, young age, multiple pregnancy, molar pregnancy, hyperthyroidism, previously suffered with motion sickness. **(1 mark for each, max 3 marks)**
3. Urine dipstick looking for presence of ketones. This suggests starvation and ketosis. **(1)**
4. U&Es (assess kidney function/dehydration), TFTs (assess hyperthyroid states), LFTs, ABG, FBC. **(1)**
5. Thiamine to prevent Wernicke's encephalopathy. **(2)**
6. Low molecular weight heparin, intravenous fluids, anti-emetics, total parenteral nutrition, steroids. **(1)**
7. Molar pregnancy. **(1)**

Hyperemesis gravidarum is nausea and vomiting in pregnancy enough to cause admission due to dehydration and possible electrolyte disturbance. An important investigation is to look for ketones in the urine, as this will give a good indication of whether the patient is severely dehydrated. There is argument over the use of anti-emetics as it is thought that the vomiting is mostly related to the circulating levels of pregnancy hormones such as βhCG. The mainstay of management is to rule out predisposing causes (the most important of which is molar pregnancy) and give supportive care with intravenous fluids. Steroids and total parenteral nutrition are last-resort options. In extreme cases, it can cause Wernicke's encephalopathy, which is a triad of ataxia, ophthalmoplegia and confusion more commonly seen in alcoholic patients.

# A³

1. Missed miscarriage: the foetus is dead but is retained in utero.

   Incomplete miscarriage: some tissue is expelled, yet some is maintained in utero.

   Inevitable miscarriage: the cervix is dilated, but the products of conception have not been expelled yet. **(3 marks)**
2. Full blood count, group and save, serum βhCG. **(2)**
3. Surgical evacuation with dilatation and curettage or suction curette, medical treatment with misoprostol and mifepristone, expectant management. **(1 mark for each, max 2 marks)**

4. Histology, karyotyping. **(1)**
5. Injury to the cervix, perforation of the uterus, scarring of the intrauterine lining (Asherman's syndrome), standard operative risks, e.g. anaesthetic risks, bleeding, infection, etc. **(1 mark for each, max 2 marks)**
6. Infection, cervical incompetence, parental chromosomal abnormality, uterine abnormalities, e.g. bicornuate uterus or large fibroids, antiphospholipid antibodies. **(1 mark for each, max 3 marks)**

Miscarriage is defined as the loss of a pregnancy before 24 weeks' gestation. Incidence is difficult to define, as pregnancies can miscarry before pregnancy is diagnosed. Presentation may be from vaginal bleeding and there may be significant blood loss and shock present. It is important to correct this and institute definitive management quickly if this is the case. Serial hCG measurement and ultrasound scanning are the main investigations of early-pregnancy vaginal bleeding with a stable patient. Indications for surgical intervention include retained products on ultrasound and persistent or profuse bleeding. Mifeprostone and misoprostol can be used to expel retained products. Stable patients can be managed expectantly and may pass products spontaneously. Second-trimester miscarriage may be due to cervical incompetence, uterine abnormality such as fibroids or maternal disease such as SLE or diabetes. Miscarriage carries psychological morbidity and as well as medical management, emotional and social support should be made available.

# A⁴

1. Dysfunctional uterine bleeding, fibroids, adenomyosis, pelvic infection, endometrial polyp, hypothyroidism, endometrial carcinoma, coagulopathy. **(1 mark for each, max 3 marks)**
2. Pelvic ultrasound, endometrial sampling, hysteroscopy. **(1 mark for each, max 2 marks)**
3. Current or history of venous thromboembolism, oestrogen-dependent cancer, current or history of stroke or coronary artery disease, benign or malignant liver tumours, migraine, heavy smoker over 35. **(1 mark for each, max 2 marks)**
4. Tranexamic acid. **(1)**
5. Insertion of mirena coil, endometrial resection/ablation. **(2)**

6. Bleeding, infection, venous thromboembolism, damage to surrounding organs (e.g. bowel, bladder, ureter), sexual dysfunction. **(1 mark for each, max 2 marks)**

7. Endometrial carcinoma. **(1)**

Menorrhagia is a common indication for hysterectomy in the UK. It is defined as increased menstrual blood flow > 80 ml/cycle. Women present when increased loss is interfering with their life or causing significant blood loss to cause anaemia. Causes are many and should be ruled out before giving a diagnosis of dysfunctional uterine bleeding, which occurs at extremes of reproductive age. Other diagnoses include polyps, fibroids, endometriosis, pelvic infections, endometrial carcinoma and adeno-myosis. Bleeding may be made worse by hypothyroidism or inherited or acquired bleeding tendencies. Investigation includes ultrasound, full blood count and endometrial sampling. Hysteroscopy with curettage can be performed to obtain histological samples. Medications include tranexamic acid if no history of VTE. Younger non-smokers may benefit from the combined oral contraceptive pill. Progesterone-containing IUCDs such as mirena can control bleeding, as can endometrial abla-tion. However, some women who have finished their families opt for hysterectomy.

# A⁵

1. Human papilloma virus. **(1)**
2. High parity, multiple sexual partners, early first intercourse, immunosupression, other STIs, smoking. **(1 mark for each, max 2 marks)**
3. Colposcopy. **(1)**
4. It is growth of endocervical columnar epithelium outside of the external os. It appears red in comparison to squamous epithelium. **(1)**
5. COCP use, pregnancy. **(1)**
6. Cervical intraepithelial neoplasia is a premalignant condition where abnormally dividing cells have not invaded below the basement membrane; in CIN III, abnormal cells occupy a full three thirds of epithelium. **(2)**
7. Large loop excision of the transition zone (LLETZ). **(1)**

8. Squamous cell, adenocarcinoma. **(2)**
9. CT scanning. **(1)**

Cervical carcinoma deaths still number around 1000 per year, but this has fallen since the introduction of the cervical cancer screening programme. With a long latent phase and a large benefit from early treatment, a screening programme is beneficial. Regular cervical smears from the age of 25 look for abnormal cells that suggest cervical intraepithelial neoplasia (CIN), which is a premalignant condition. Human papilloma virus types 16, 18 and 33 are all associated with cervical cancer. As this is a sexually transmitted disease, risk factors include early first intercourse and multiple sexual partners. Dyskaryotic smears should be referred for colposcopy and biopsy. CIN can be treated with cryotherapy, laser therapy or large loop excision of the transition zone (LLETZ). Invasive disease can present as intermenstrual or post-coital bleeding, and is treated according to its stage. Stage I cancers can be treated with radical hysterectomy and pelvic lymphadenectomy. Higher stages are treated with radiotherapy and platinum-based chemotherapy.

## A⁶

1. Ovarian cyst rupture, ovarian cyst haemorrhage, ectopic pregnancy, ovarian torsion. **(2)**
2. Pelvic ultrasound, urine βhCG. **(2)**
3. Sudden-onset severe lower abdominal pain, possibly with peritonism. This arises when a small cyst rotates on a free pedicle and restricts its blood supply, causing potential ovarian necrosis. **(2)**
4. Dermoid cyst. **(1)**
5. Derived from primitive germ cells which can differentiate into any body tissue, e.g. hair, teeth, sebaceous material, bone, etc. **(1)**
6. Dermoid cysts have a very low risk of being malignant. **(1)**
7. Nulliparity, infertility, family history, early menarche, late menopause, Caucasian. **(2)**
8. *BRCA1* or *BRCA2*. **(1)**
9. Ca-125, alpha-fetoprotein. **(1)**

Ovarian masses are frequently found in asymptomatic women as an incidental finding as they are very prevalent. They also may present to the emergency department as an acute abdomen with complications such as cyst rupture, haemorrhage or torsion. Benign tumours may be functional cysts from persistent follicles or corpus luteum, endometriomas, theca-lutein cysts, epithelial cysts or dermoid cysts. Malignant tumours are rarer but carry a poor outcome, with a 5-year survival rate of around 20%–75%, but this varies widely according to stage. Masses may be palpable on examination, and malignant tumours can cause ascites. Transvaginal ultrasound scanning can confirm presence of cystic or solid masses, and tumours can be removed by laparoscopy or open surgery. One particular tumour type, dermoid cysts, are mature teratomas and contain germ cells that may have differentiated into another tissue such as skin, hair or teeth.

# A⁷

1. The presence and development of endometrial tissue outside of the endometrial cavity. **(1)**
2. Ovary, rectovaginal pouch, uterosacral ligaments, pelvic peritoneum, umbilicus, lower abdominal scars, lung. **(1 mark for each, max 2 marks)**
3. Age, long duration of IUCD use, smoking, positive family history. **(1)**
4. Chronic pelvic pain, may be cyclical radiating to legs, dyspareunia, dysuria, pain on defecation, cyclical rectal bleeding, cyclical diarrhoea, cyclical haematuria. **(1 mark for each, max 2 marks)**
5. Adenomyosis. **(1)**
6. Infertility, pelvic adhesions, ruptured cysts, bowel obstruction, chronic pelvic pain. **(1 mark for each, max 2 marks)**
7. Fixed, retroverted uterus, uterosacral ligament nodules, tender uterus, enlarged ovaries, visible lesions in vagina or on cervix. **(1 mark for each, max 2 marks)**
8. Analgesia/NSAIDs, COCP to supress ovulation, progesterone-only pill (POP), mirena (levornogestrel-containing intrauterine device), GnRH agonists. **(1 mark for each, max 2 marks)**
9. Laparoscopy with excision/ablation of endometrial deposits; total hysterectomy + bilateral salpingo-oophorectomy. **(1 mark for each, max 2 marks)**

Endometriosis is the presence of endometrial glandular tissue outside of the uterine cavity. Common sites are ovary, rectovesical pouch, uterosacral ligaments and pelvic peritoneum. If the tissue is found in the uterine smooth muscle, it is termed adenomyosis. Pathological features arise as the deposits are under hormonal control, so they bleed during menstruation. Bleeding provokes inflammation, which leads to adhesions and chronic pain. Symptoms include dysmenorrhoea, chronic pelvic pain, subfertility and dyspareunia. Bowel and bladder symptoms may also be present. Examination findings include fixed tender retroverted uterus with uterosacral ligament nodules. Non-steroidal analgesia can help the pain, but persistent pain may benefit from ovulation suppression using combined pill, hormone-releasing IUCDs, or GnRH agonists. Surgical treatment includes laparoscopy and excision or ablation of deposits or, if no wishes for fertility, a hysterectomy and bilateral salpingo-oophorectomy.

# A⁸

1. Primary infertility is where the couple have never been able to conceive; secondary infertility is where the couple have achieved conception in the past. **(1)**
2. Anovulation (PCOS, chemotherapy, hyperprolactinaemia), tubal occlusion (e.g. PID/previous tubal ligation), uterine abnormality, endometriosis, hostile cervical mucus. **(3)**
3. Stop smoking, prepregnancy vitamins, weight loss, avoid alcohol. **(1 mark for each, max 2 marks)**
4. Day 21 progesterone of a 28-day cycle, FSH/LH, estradiol, prolactin. **(1 mark for each, max 2 marks)**
5. Hysterosalpingogram, laparoscopy and dye test. **(1 mark for each, max 1 mark)**
6. Hirsutism, acne, male pattern baldness, amenorrhoea, central obesity, infertility, symptoms of diabetes, acanthosis nigricans. **(1 mark for each, max 2 marks)**
7. Metformin, clomiphene citrate, gonadotrophins. **(1 mark for each, max 2 marks)**

Subfertility is an increasingly common reason for referral to gynaecology. Factors from both partners may be involved in the process, and treatment should involve both partners. More than 90% of couples having regular intercourse will conceive within 2 years. Broad causes of subfertility are anovulatory (commonly PCOS), male factors, tubal factors, sexual dysfunction or chromosomal abnormalities. Initial consultation encourages a healthy lifestyle with preconception folic acid and smoking cessation.

Day 21 progesterone can be checked to ensure patient is ovulating. Other investigations include TFTs, LH (for PCOS), prolactin, FSH, semen analysis and pelvic ultrasound. More invasive investigations are laparoscopy with dye testing to check tubal patency. Treatments target the cause with ovulation induction, clomifene being the treatment of choice for PCOS and anovulation, and hysteroscopic adhesiolysis for tubal factors. For some couples, assisted conception with intrauterine insemination or in vitro fertilisation is an option. Psychological effects of remaining childless should not be underestimated.

## A⁹

1. Laparoscopic tubal ligation:
   - advantages – highly effective, permanent, cheaper if used over a long period of time, a slightly decreased risk of ovarian cancer
   - disadvantages – abdominal surgery general anaesthetic carries associated morbidity and mortality, very difficult if not impossible to reverse.

   Hormone-releasing intrauterine contraceptive device:
   - advantages – long-term contraception (up to 5 years), no ongoing tablets, low associated mortality, associated reduction in menstrual bleeding
   - disadvantages – insertion may be unacceptable to patient, small risk of ectopic pregnancy and PID, may be expelled in distorted or nulliparous uteruses, progestogenic side effects (acne, low mood, weight gain, bloating). **(1 mark for each, max 4 marks)**

2. Pregnancy, sexually transmitted infection, cancer of ovary, cancer of endometrium, cervical cancer, trophoblastic disease. **(1 mark for each, max 2 marks)**

3. Cervical shock causes a vasovagal reaction with reflex bradycardia. **(1)**

4. Acute pelvic infection (endometritis/salpingitis) leading to pelvic inflammatory disease due to insertion of an IUCD. **(1)**

5. *Chlamydia trachomatis*, *Neisseria gonorrhoeae*, standard vaginal flora, streptococcal, *Mycobacterium tuberculosis*, Gram-negative organisms from GI tract, e.g. *E. coli*, *Trichomonas vaginalis*. **(1 mark for each, max 2 marks)**

6. IV antibiotics, e.g. ceftriaxone and doxycycline +/– metronidazole. **(1)**
7. Chronic salpingitis with menorrhagia, dyspareunia and dysmenorrhoea, formation of tubo-ovarian abscess, infertility, ectopic pregnancy, chronic pelvic pain. **(2)**

Contraception is an important topic which enables women to control their childbearing capacity and empowers them to make their own choices. There are multiple methods, with different methods suiting different women. The cost in time and money to provide contraceptive services may be more beneficial than the risks of an unwanted or dangerous pregnancy. Natural methods such as the rhythm method require strong discipline and have high failure rates, but are free from any intervention. Barrier methods such as condoms are also free from hormones and have the added protection from transmitting most STIs; however, this is unacceptable to some couples in terms of sexual function. Hormonal medications such as the COCP are effective, but require discipline and are not without side effects and risks such as DVT. Progesterone preparations in the form of depot injection, implants and IUCDs are further options to be explored. Finally, surgical treatments such as tubal ligation and vasectomy provide permanent contraception, so the decision to undertake these methods should not be made lightly.

# A¹⁰

1. Atrophic vaginitis, endometrial hyperplasia, endometrial polyps, cervical polyps, carcinoma of vagina or cervix, ovarian cancer, vaginal trauma, infection. **(1 mark for each, max 2 marks)**
2. Adenocarcinoma. **(1)**
3. Obesity, nulliparity, unopposed oestrogen treatment, late menopause, previous pelvic radiation, tamoxifen, polycystic ovaries, family history. **(1 mark for each, max 2 marks)**
4. Transvaginal ultrasound scan of pelvis. **(1)**
5. Radical hysterectomy and bilateral salpingo-oophorectomy. **(1)**
6. External beam radiotherapy, high-dose medroxyprogesterone acetate, chemotherapy. **(1 mark for each, max 2 marks)**
7. Inguinal lymph nodes, lung, bone, supraclavicular lymph node, vagina, liver, peritoneum. **(1 mark for each, max 2 marks)**

Post-menopausal bleeding should prompt referral for investigation as endometrial carcinoma is a possible diagnosis. It arises from glandular endometrium which has been subjected to oestrogen without opposing progesterone. Risk factors therefore reflect states of increased exposure to oestrogen, such as obesity, nulliparity and late menopause. Other than post-menopausal bleeding, endometrial carcinoma may present as abnormal glandular cells on routine cervical smear tests. Tumours arise in the uterine endometrium and grow into the myometrium, cervix, vagina or peritoneum. Diagnosis is aided by transvaginal ultrasound, which reveals thickened endometrium. Endometrial sampling is then used to obtain tissue for a histological diagnosis. Should tissue be insufficient from endometrial sampling, hysteroscopy, dilatation and curettage can be used to obtain tissue. Treatment depends on the stage, with cancer localised to the uterus and cervix amenable to radical hysterectomy. More advanced tumours can be treated with pre-operative/post-operative radiotherapy, or radium brachytherapy. High-dose progesterone can be used to downstage a tumour. Extension outside the pelvis may be treated with systemic chemotherapy.

# Elderly care

1.  Drop in systolic BP by > 20 mmHg and/or drop in diastolic BP by > 10 mmHg within the first 10 minutes of standing. **(1)**
2.  Antihypertensive agents. **(1)**
3.  Numerous other medications (e.g. nitrates, diuretics, many antidepressant agents), excessive alcohol consumption, hypovolaemia (haemorrhage, dehydration, diarrhoea, Addison's), primary autonomic failure (e.g. Parkinson's disease, multiple system atrophy), secondary autonomic failure, e.g. diabetic neuropathy. **(1 mark for each, max 2 marks)**
4.  Full-length compression hosiery, education on recognising symptoms and taking action, high-salt diet, bed tilt. **(1 mark for each, max 2 marks)**
5.  Fludrocortisone, midodrine. **(1 mark for each, max 2 marks)**
6.  Arthritis, reduced cognition, polypharmacy, reduced visual input, reduced muscle strength, reduced proprioception, increased reaction time. **(1 mark for each, max 2 marks)**

Falls are common in the elderly, and the number of causes is vast. Arthritis, reduced cognition, polypharmacy, reduced visual input, reduced muscle strength, reduced proprioception and an increased reaction time all contribute to the increased risk of falling. As a junior doctor, you will be asked to assess numerous patients who have been admitted with falls, or who have fallen during their admission. It is important to take a full history to establish the mechanism of the fall, whether consciousness was lost, what injuries have been sustained, etc. A collateral history from someone who witnessed the fall can be extremely helpful. Postural hypotension is a fall in blood pressure on standing. Antihypertensives are commonly responsible, and stopping them often resolves the problem. However, in many cases no cause will be found. Non-pharmacological measures should be tried first, such as full-length compression hosiery, tilting the bed so it is more upright and increasing salt in the diet. Fludrocortisone is a synthetic mineralocorticoid and acts to increase the intravascular volume, hence raising the blood pressure. Midodrine is a locally acting vascular bed vasoconstrictor, and is contraindicated in those with peripheral vascular disease and coronary artery disease.

# A²

1. A syndrome of clouding of consciousness, disorientation, perceptual impairment and changes in affect and behaviour. **(2 marks for similar answer)**
2. Confusion Assessment Method (CAM). **(1)**
3. Iatrogenic (e.g. steroids, opioids), metabolic (e.g. renal failure, hepatic failure, hypoglycaemia), electrolyte imbalance (e.g. hyponatraemia, hypernatraemia, hypocalcaemia), severe pain. **(1 mark for each, max 3 marks)**
4. Coliforms, e.g. *E. coli*. **(1)**
5. Inhibit cell wall synthesis. **(1)**
6. Beta-lactamase production (breaks down the beta-lactam ring). **(1)**
7. Beta-lactamase inhibitors. **(1)**

Delirium, or acute confusional state, is commonly seen in elderly patients admitted to hospital and is characterised by fluctuating levels of consciousness. Infections, particularly UTIs, are often responsible for delirium. Other causes include metabolic disturbance, steroids and pain. Differentiating between delirium and dementia can be challenging; dementia occurs in clear consciousness. The Confusion Assessment Method can be used to differentiate between the two, and a diagnosis of delirium requires features one and two, as well as either feature three or four. Patients with delirium are often distressed, and simple management should include trying to reduce this and helping to reorientate them. Family members can often be very useful at helping with this. As a junior doctor, you will regularly be called to the elderly care wards overnight to consider night sedation for patients with delirium, as they are often very difficult for nursing staff to manage. These patients are often at an increased risk of falls, and sedatives will increase that risk, particularly if wandering is a feature of their delirium. This should be considered prior to prescribing night sedation.

# A³

1. Personality change, behavioural change, inattention, changes in mood, language/communication deficits, loss of judgement, disorientation. **(1 mark for each, max 2 marks)**
2. Vascular dementia, Lewy body dementia. **(1 mark for each, max 2 marks)**
3. $B_{12}$ deficiency, thiamine deficiency, normal pressure hydrocephalus, uraemia, hypothyroidism, hypoglycaemia. **(1 mark for each, max 2 marks)**
4. Cortical atrophy, ventricular enlargement, hippocampal atrophy. **(1 mark for each, max 2 marks)**
5. Anticholinergics, e.g. donepezil, rivastigmine. **(1)**
6. Inhibition of acetylcholinesterase; therefore, less acetycholine is broken down, and hence more is available at the synapse. **(1 mark for adequate explanation)**

Dementia is a syndrome of acquired global impairment of higher mental functions that occurs in clear consciousness. It is normally progressive and irreversible, although there are some reversible causes, such as $B_{12}$ deficiency, thiamine deficiency and hypothyroidism. It is commonly in the elderly population. Alzheimer's disease is the commonest form of dementia and typically presents over a number of years with progressive memory loss. Vascular dementia is a result of cerebrovascular disease, and the risk factors are the same as those for cardiovascular disease. Its progression is typically described as being step-wise. Patients with Lewy body dementia tend to have a fluctuating level of dementia and numerous delirium-like phases. Visual hallucinations are common in this form of dementia, as are signs of Parkinsonism.

# A⁴

1. Stress incontinence. **(1)**
2. Pelvic floor muscles. **(1)**
3. Diuretics (e.g. furosemide, bumetanide, bendroflumethiazide), sedative (e.g. opiates, antipsychotics). **(1 mark for any of above)**
4. Pregnancy, childbirth, obesity, chronic constipation, chronic cough, post-menopause (due to reduced oestrogen). **(½ a mark for each, max 1 mark)**
5. Anticholinergics (e.g. tolterodine, oxybutynin), NSAIDs (e.g. naproxen, diclofenac, ibuprofen). **(1 mark for any of above)**

6. Pelvic floor exercises, avoid caffeine, avoid/stop smoking, weight loss (if appropriate). **(1 mark for each, max 2 marks)**

7. Duloxetine is an SNRI, so inhibits the reuptake of noradrenaline (NA) at the synapse, meaning there is increased NA available, and this increases the tone of the internal urethral sphincter. **(2 marks for satisfactory explanation)**

8. ACE inhibitor (next appropriate management step according to NICE guidelines, dry cough is a side effect which may exacerbate stress incontinence). **(1)**

Incontinence is considered one of the 'geriatric giants'. Stress incontinence is a common problem in older women, and it often causes the patient significant distress and embarrassment. Weakness of the pelvic floor is responsible for stress incontinence, and is commonly caused by the weight of the uterus during pregnancy and stretching of the muscles during pregnancy. Increasing the tone of pelvic floor muscles should be encouraged, and numerous programmes explaining how to do this, how often and for how long are advised by physiotherapists. Conservative management also includes addressing exacerbating factors, such as obesity, smoking and drinking large volumes of caffeine. Duloxetine is given to some patients. The internal urethral sphincter is under autononomic control, and increasing the NA at the synapse increases sympathetic activity and increases its tone. Surgical options include referral to a urogynaecologist for consideration of tension-free vaginal tapes/sling procedures.

# A5

1. $ABCD^2$ score. **(1)**

2. Age, blood pressure, clinical features, duration, diabetes. **(1 mark for each, max 3 marks)**

3. Carotid endarterectomy. **(1)**

4. Hypertension, smoking, hypercholesterolaemia, diabetes, AF, previous TIA, antiphospholipid syndrome, polycythaemia. **(1 mark for each, max 3 marks)**

5. Inhibits the reductase enzyme responsible for regeneration of active vitamin K, hence inhibiting the production of vitamin K-dependent clotting factors (II, VII, IX, X). **(2 marks for reasonable explanation)**

Transient ischaemic attacks (TIAs) are usually caused by emboli, and are characterised by focal neurology signs and symptoms that resolve within 24 hours. If symptoms last longer than this, the diagnosis is stroke. TIAs commonly precede a larger event, and addressing risk factors early may prevent this. The $ABCD^2$ score has been developed to determine the immediate risk of a stroke following a TIA. The components are age ($< 60 = 0$, $\geq 60 = 1$), blood pressure ($\geq 140$ systolic or $\geq 90 = 1$), clinical features (unilateral weakness = 2, speech disturbance without weakness = 1), duration of symptoms ($\geq 60$ minutes = 2, 10–59 minutes = 1, $< 10$ minutes = 0) and whether or not the patient is diabetic (diabetes = 1). Those with a score of 0–3 are deemed at low risk, those scoring 4–5 have a moderate risk and those scoring 6–7 are at high risk. Treatment should be directed at managing cardiovascular risk factors, anticoagulation and investigation of the carotid arteries with doppler USS. If there is significant stenosis, carotid endarterectomy may be appropriate.

## A⁶

1. Internal carotid artery. **(1)**
2. Circle of Willis. **(1)**
3. Left total anterior circulation infarct (TACI). **(1 mark for left, 1 mark for TAC, 1 mark for infarct)**
4. Alteplase. **(1)**
5. Age < 18 or > 80, haemorrhagic stroke, suspected subarachnoid haemorrhage, active bleeding, major surgery within 14 days, GI bleed within last 21 days, thrombocytopenia $< 100 \times 10^9$/L, pregnancy, systolic BP > 185, diastolic BP > 110, previous intracranial haemorrhage, neurosurgery within last 3 months, recent lumbar puncture, hypoglycaemia. **(1 mark for each, max 4 marks)**

Strokes are commonly seen in the elderly population, and are often terminal events. The risk factors for cerebrovascular disease are the same as those for cardiovascular disease, such as hypertension, diabetes, hypercholesterolaemia and smoking. Patients with atrial fibrillation are also at an increased risk of stroke due to the formation of thrombus in the left atrium and subsequent embolisation to the cerebral arteries. The arterial network in the brain is called the Circle of Willis. The anterior communicating artery links the two anterior cerebral arteries, and the posterior communicating arteries link the internal carotid arteries to the posterior cerebral arteries. This allows redistribution of blood flow within the brain if it has been compromised.

# A⁷

1. Post-menopausal women, low BMI, depot progesterone, increasing age, malnutrition, smoking, positive paternal history, alcohol excess, various medical condition (e.g. Cushing's, RA, chronic kidney disease), long-term corticosteroids. (½ **a mark for each, max 2 marks**)

2. Hip, distal radius, proximal humerus, vertebrae. (**1 mark for each, max 3 marks**)

3. T-score: the number of standard deviations of the patient's bone mineral density value is below that of an average young adult

   Z-score: the number of standard deviations the patient's bone mineral density value is below that of a population matched for age, gender, ethnicity, etc. (**1 mark for each**)

4. Swallow whole, take in fasting state, wash down with plenty of water, remain upright for 30 minutes after taking the tablet, avoid food and drink for 30 minutes after taking the tablet. (**1 mark for each, max 2 marks**)

5. Abdominal pain, dyspepsia, nausea, abdominal distension, oesophageal ulceration, upper GI bleed. (**1 mark for each, max 2 marks**)

Osteoporosis is a reduced bone mineral density. This leaves the bone vulnerable to fracture. Common sites for osteoporotic fractures are the hip, proximal humerus, distal radius, pubic ramus and vertebrae. Major risk factors for the development of osteoporosis include post-menopausal women, increasing age, malnutrition, smoking, chronic alcohol excess and long-term steroids. Secondary prevention includes replenishing $Ca2+$ and vitamin D stores, and using bisphosphonates. NICE recommends secondary prevention in all those > 75 with evidence of a fragility fracture. In those < 75, NICE states they should be further investigated with a dual-energy X-ray absoptiometry (DEXA) scan. The T-score compares the patient's bone mineral density with that of an average young male, and if the score is < –2.5, osteoporosis is diagnosed.

# A⁸

1. Urinary Bence Jones protein, serum electrophoresis. **(1 mark for each, max 2 marks)**
2. Lytic lesions. **(1)**
3. Spinal cord compression. **(1)**
4. Dexamethasone. **(1)**
5. MRI spine. **(1)**
6. Radiotherapy, surgical decompression. **(1 mark for each, max 2 marks)**
7. Hypercalcaemia, acute kidney injury, hyperviscosity, recurrent bacterial infections/neutropenia, anaemia, thrombocytopenia. **(1 mark for each, max 2 marks)**

Myeloma is a malignancy of plasma cells. Large proportions of identical immunoglobulins (Igs) are produced by a single clone of plasma cells, and these are known as monoclonal paraproteins. In the majority of cases, these are IgG. Electrophoresis of the serum detects these as a monoclonal band. Light chains from these Igs may be excreted in the urine, and these are known as Bence Jones proteins. Myeloma causes destruction of bone, causing pain, hypercalcaemia and pathological fractures. Radiographs typically reveal lytic lesions. Renal impairment may also be seen in patients with myeloma, and this is caused by a number of factors, including hypercalcaemia, deposition of light chains in the tubules, NSAIDs and amyloid deposition. Bone marrow infiltration can lead to its suppression, and cause anaemia, thrombocytopenia and neutropenia. This neutropenia may leave patients vulnerable to infections. Chemotherapy is often the treatment of choice. Allogeneic transplantation may be used in younger patients as it offers a cure. However, it also carries a significant risk of mortality.

# A⁹

1. Degeneration of dopaminergic neurones within the substantia nigra, leading to increased muscle activity. **(1)**
2. Rigidity (cog-wheeling, lead-pipe rigidity), bradykinesia. **(1 mark for each, max 2 marks)**
3. Mask-like face, postural/orthostatic hypotension, festinating gait, micrographia, drooling, monotonous speech. **(1 mark for each, max 2 marks)**

4. Drug-induced Parkinsonism (e.g. antipsychotics), Lewy body dementia, Shy–Drager syndrome, multiple system atrophy, vascular disease. **(1 mark for each, max 2 marks)**

5. They are peripheral decarboxylase inhibitors, preventing L-dopa from being broken down outside the CNS. **(1)**

6. It becomes gradually ineffective over many years; therefore, held until necessary. **(1)**

7. Benign essential tremor. **(1)**

Parkinson's disease is characterised by bradykinesia, increased tone and tremor. It results from degeneration of dopaminergic neurones within the substantia nigra. Dopamine is responsible for inhibition of muscular activity, and degeneration means its inhibitory effect is less than the excitatory effect of acetylcholine. Levodopa is commonly given to patients with Parkinson's disease, but over time its effects are reduced. This leads to fluctuating responses to the drug, dyskinesia, choreiform movements and dystonias. Also, the duration of its action is reduced. For these reasons, it is often held in reserve for younger patients, and other medications are tried first. Examples of other treatments include dopamine agonist and amantidine.

## A10

1. Benign prostatic hypertrophy, prostatitis, post-prostatic biopsy, post-digital rectal examination. **(1 mark for each, max 2 marks)**

2. Raised alkaline phosphatase. **(1)**

3. Intravenous fluids, intravenous bisphosphonates. **(1 mark for each, max 2 marks)**

4. Pain (morphine), agitation (midazolam), nausea (cyclizine), respiratory tract secretions (hyoscine butylbromide/hydrobromide), dyspnoea (morphine). **(½ a mark for each symptom, ½ a mark for appropriate drug)**

The Liverpool Care Pathway (LCP) is a pathway for patients in the last days of life. It was first developed in Liverpool, but has now been adopted throughout the UK. The pathway involves information for relatives, as well as guidelines and management algorithms for medical professions and nursing staff. Most, if not all, hospitals will have specialist palliative care nurses, and they can be extremely helpful in managing difficult scenarios regarding end-of-life care. The pathway addresses the most distressing symptoms patients may develop in the last stages of life, and offers guidance on how they should be managed. Patients in pain and with dyspnoea should receive morphine, agitation is managed with midazolam, respiratory tract secretions require hyoscine and nauseous patients are given cyclizine. All medications should be given subcutaneously, and a syringe driver may be necessary if patients require the above medications regularly. In addition, all non-essential medications should be stopped. It is important to remember that palliative care is not only confined to those with cancer. The pathway suggests regular reassessment to ensure the patient is comfortable and that the correct decision has been made.

# Psychiatry

## A¹

1. Mood symptoms: irritability, euphoria, emotional lability.

   Cognitive symptoms: pressure of speech, confusion, flight of ideas, poor concentration, easily distracted.

   Behavioural symptoms: hyperactivity, reduced sleep, extravagant spending, promiscuity.

   Psychotic symptoms: delusions of grandeur, hallucinations. **(1 mark for each, max 4 marks)**

2. Feelings of invincibility lead to reckless behaviour, for example with money, leading to financial problems; hypersexuality may lead to dangerous situations and risks of unwanted pregnancy and STIs; increased use of alcohol/illicit substances comes with potential physical consequences. **(1 mark for each, max 2 marks)**

3. Amphetamines, cocaine, antidepressants, corticosteroids, procyclidine, levodopa. **(2)**

4. This means the patient has voluntarily agreed to treatment of a mental illness, and is not detained against their will. They are free to leave if they please. **(1)**

5. ECG: lithium can cause long QT syndrome.

   Thyroid function tests: baseline TFTs are needed as lithium may reduce the activity of thyroid hormones.

   Urea and electrolytes: lithium can affect renal function in overdose. **(3 marks)**

6. Suicidal ideation and history of deliberate self-harm. **(max 1 mark)**

7. Nausea, diarrhoea, vomiting, ataxia, confusion, lethargy, polyuria, seizures coma, tremor, convulsions, renal failure. **(½ a mark for each, max 1 mark)**

Bipolar affective disorder is a mood disorder characterised by periods of depression alternating with periods of elevated mood and energy levels.

Severe episodes may be complicated by psychotic symptoms, such as delusions of grandeur and hallucinations. Diagnosis is clinical, using psychiatric history taking and collateral histories from relatives. Acute presentations should have a suicide risk assessment as part of initial consultation. Most patients present in young adulthood, although it may present at any age. A manic episode may cause sufficient distress to the patient and families that hospitalisation is used. There is a strong genetic component, with many patients having a close relative with the disease. Rarely, the cause may be drug-induced or organic. Treatment centres on the halting of an acute episode with medications such as olanzapine, with follow-up maintenance treatment with lithium, valproate, carbamazepine or a combination of these. Lithium toxicity is a potentially fatal side effect of treatment. Follow-up will be long-term, with high risk of relapse.

# A²

1. Low mood, anhedonia, lasting for more than 2 weeks, change from previous functioning. **(3 marks)**
2. Poor appetite with weight loss (5% of more of body weight in a month), early morning wakening, diurnal mood variation, psychomotor retardation, decrease in sexual function, inability to concentrate, feelings of worthlessness/guilt/self-reproach, thoughts of death or suicide, delusions or hallucinations of death or worthlessness. **(½ a mark each, max 2 marks)**
3. A suicide risk assessment and an assessment of risk to others. **(1)**
4. Diagnostic, monitoring of symptoms, research. **(1 mark for each, max 2 marks)**
5. Significant variation of scores between different populations or cultures; they are only validated in hospitals, not general population. **(1 mark for each, max 2 marks)**
6. Psychotherapy (e.g CBT), antidepressant medications, e.g. SSRIs, herbal remedies (e.g. St John's wort), ECT (if severe with delusions, hallucinations needing admission). **(1 mark for each, max 2 marks)**
7. Chronic diseases: cancer, diabetes, cardiac failure, COPD, etc.

   Other mental illnesses: bipolar disorder, schizophrenia, etc.

   Medical conditions: hypothyroidism, Addison's, perimenopausal. **(1 mark for each, max 2 marks)**

8. Vegetative symptoms: weight increase, increase of appetite, hypersomnolence.

   Catatonic symptoms: leaden limbs, social impairment.

   Mood: mood may lighten with positive events. **(max 1 mark)**

Major depression is a common psychiatric illness affecting all levels of society. It is distinguished from general feelings of depression by physical symptoms such as sleep difficulty, loss of appetite, anhedonia and sometimes suicidal ideation. Other physical symptoms include early morning wakening, sexual dysfunction and psychomotor retardation. Depression is extremely common in patients with chronic debilitating illness and is often overlooked in clinical assessment. There is a significant risk of suicide, and all patients should be assessed for suicidal ideation. Treatment is varied and long-term, ranging from psychological interventions such as cognitive behavioural therapy to antidepressants, antipsychotics and in severe cases electroconvulsive therapy. Admission should be considered in those patients with high suicidal drive or isolated social circumstances.

## A³

1. Delirium is an acute (hours/days) and fluctuating type of altered consciousness, specifically with confusion and disorientation, made worse by the fact that the ability to recall memories is lost. Delirium is a syndrome with an organic origin.

   Dementia is a chronic disorder caused by a disease of the brain. Memory is also affected, but parts of the brain controlling personality and reasoning are often affected by dementia. **(2)**

2. Infection: UTI, LRTI, wound infection, cellulitis, etc.

   Metabolic: hypoxia, hypoglycaemia, dehydration causing electrolyte imbalance.

   Drug-induced: opioids, benzodiazepines, anticholinergic, alcohol, anaesthetics, illicit drugs, psychotropic medications, digoxin, antiepileptics.

   Drug withdrawal including alcohol.

   Neurological: head trauma, intracranial bleeding, mass, infection, stroke, epilepsy.

Pain: e.g. urinary retention, constipation.

Sensory disturbance: e.g. missing glasses or hearing aids. **(½ a mark each, max 2 marks)**

3. Alzheimer's dementia, vascular dementia, Lewy body dementia, Parkinson's dementia, Huntington's disease, HIV dementia, alcoholic dementia. Rarer causes: maple syrup urine disease, CJD. **(½ a mark each, max 2 marks)**

4. Moderately lit and quiet room, ideally easily monitored by nurses.

   Ensure familiar nursing staff, and calming non-aggressive voice to orientate the patient.

   Optimise sensory/communication function, e.g. hearing aids, interpreters, false teeth, glasses.

   'Specialing' patient with one-to-one caregiver. **(1 mark for each, max 2 marks)**

5. Increased confusion, increased fall risk, respiratory depression and hypotension; sedation may make history-taking and examination more difficult. **(1 mark for each, max 2 marks)**

6. Physiotherapist, occupational therapist, social worker, pharmacist, ward nursing staff, community and district nursing staff. **(½ a mark each, max 2 marks)**

7. Orientation to time: from broad to narrow.

   Orientation to place: from broad to narrow.

   Attention and calculation: serial sevens (100 − 7, etc.).

   Language/recall: name objects and remember previous address.

   Spatial awareness/complex demands: drawing.

   Registration. **(½ a mark each, max 1 mark)**

Delirium is a common sight on acute medical and surgical wards. Delirium is an organic condition characterised by an impaired consciousness over the course of hours and days. The causes are many, including infection, metabolic disturbance, hypoxia, sedative medications and sensory impairment. Delirium should be differentiated from anxiety by history and dementia by time of onset. Delirium can occur in the setting of a chronic cognitive impairment such as Alzheimer's dementia, and indeed these patients are more at risk, being in new and distressing environments. Treatment should focus on the cause, and this should be investigated with FBC, U&E, glucose, $PaO_2$, microbiology cultures and appropriate imaging. In the interim patients should be nursed in a calm environment, and non-pharmacological treatments should be employed. In extreme circumstances, medications such as haloperidol or lorazepam can be used to treat agitation. Delirium is a reversible process, but may complicate hospital stays and increase morbidity and mortality.

# A⁴

1. Men: 21 per week and not regularly drinking more than 3–4 units of alcohol per day.

   Women: 14 units per week and not regularly drinking more than 2–3 units per day. **(1)**

2. Continued drinking harms a person physically, mentally, socially or financially. For example, being made unemployed, ending relationships or getting into debt. **(1)**

3. Attempted and failure of abstinence, compulsion to drink, narrowing of drinking repertoire, increased tolerance to alcohol, alcohol is priority over other aspects of life, physical withdrawal when alcohol is stopped. **(2)**

4. Self-directed therapy such as slow weaning needs patient commitment to slow treatment, group psychotherapy and self-help, e.g. Alcoholics Anonymous, medical therapy, e.g disulfuram, acomprosate, education/counselling and admission for detox involving a sliding-scale dose of a benzodiazepine. **(2)**

5. Confusion and irritability, autonomic instability (fever, tachycardia, hypotension), tremor, visual or tactile hallucinations. **(½ a mark for each, max 2 marks)**

6. To prevent Wernicke's encephalopathy. **(1)**

7. Liver: fatty liver, hepatitis, cirrhosis (48% 5-year survival if drinking continues).

   CNS: cognitive dysfunction, seizures, ataxia, peripheral neuropathy.

   CVS: hypertension, strokes, cardiomyopathy.

GI tract: peptic ulcers, pancreatitis, oesophageal varices. (½ **a mark for each, max 2 marks)**

8. Disulfuram blocks acetaldehyde dehydrogenase, which is an intermediate in the breakdown of alcohol. When alcohol is ingested, acetaldehyde cannot be broken down into acetic acid, so builds up and causes unpleasant effects, such as vomiting, tachycardia, facial flushing, headache and shortness of breath. This causes a learnt aversion to alcohol through these unpleasant symptoms. **(1)**

Alcoholism is where someone's drinking leads to harm in their work or social lives. It pervades all layers of society and can manifest itself as binge drinking or regular high daily intakes. Other psychiatric diagnoses may be present and denial is a feature, so collateral history taking is important. Long-term physical effects include hepatitis, liver cirrhosis, cognitive deficits, peptic ulcers and anaemia. Withdrawal from alcohol can occur if there is a period of abstinence following long-term alcohol consumption. Signs include tremor, autonomic instability, confusion, seizures and hallucinations. This can be treated with a weaning dose of benzodiazepine medication. Long-term alcohol abuse can be treated with self-help, group therapy and developing strategies to avoid situations where alcohol can be consumed. Medications such as disulfuram act by causing severe unpleasant side effects in small ingestions of alcohol and should be used with caution.

## A5

1. Genetic predisposition and family history; male sex; obstetric/prenatal events, e.g. low birth weight, perinatal infections; cannabis use; Asian/African populations; poor social situation, such as inner-city residents or homelessness. **(2)**

2. Breaks in thought processes, incoherent or irrelevant speech, knight's move thinking, neologisms and odd logic. **(1)**

3. Thought broadcast: the feeling that people can overhear one's thoughts.

   Delusions: a false held belief with strong conviction in spite of evidence against it, not in keeping with a patient's social and cultural background. These may be persecutory, delusions of grandeur or of control.

Second-person auditory hallucinations: a perception of sound in the absence of an external stimulus. The voice in second-person hallucinations is perceived as talking straight to the person experiencing it. **(3)**

4. Apathy, reduced speech, blunted affect, social withdrawal. **(1)**
5. Inform staff members where you are, be closer to the door than the patient, calming speech and open body language, consider pharmacological sedation of the patient. **(1)**
6. Fasting blood sugar: many antipsychotics can cause diabetes in the long term.

   Weight and BP: antipsychotics can cause weight gain and hypertension in the long term, so need a baseline and 6-monthly monitoring. **(2)**
7. Antipsychotics are dopamine-2 receptor antagonists. Prolactin release from lactotrophs is inhibited by dopamine released from the hypothalamus. Therefore, when this inhibition is lifted, prolactin release is increased. **(1)**
8. An acute dystonic reaction secondary to antipsychotic medications. **(1)** Dopamine from the substantia nigra helps coordinate movement. When this dopamine is blocked, Parkinsonism symptoms can occur. **(1)**
9. There is a small risk of agranulocytosis associated with clozapine. **(1)**

Schizophrenia is a common psychiatric condition which often presents in late teens and early 20s. Psychosis with auditory hallucinations, delusions and thought disorder may occur with negative symptoms such as apathy, blunted affect, self-neglect and cognitive impairment. Symptoms include thought insertion, deletion or broadcast, second- or third-person hallucinations, catatonic behaviour and incongruous thoughts. The prevalence is about three in 1000. Susceptibility genes exist but aren't exclusive as a cause. Other theories include trigger factors such as early cannabis use or certain prenatal conditions, e.g. preterm birth. Studies in patients using MRI/CT show brains of schizophrenics tend to have larger ventricles and reduced frontal lobes. Social factors such as deprivation and being in a migrant population are also associated with schizophrenia. Antipsychotic medications are dopamine antagonists which help to manage psychotic symptoms. Care plans can involve depot antipsychotics on a fortnightly basis to help ensure compliance with therapy.

# A⁶

1.  Emotionally unstable (borderline) personality disorder (Cluster B – dramatic). **(1)**
2.  'A mental disorder': Any disorder or disability of the mind causing distress to the patient. **(1)**
3.  Section 2: admission for assessment lasts 28 days.

    Section 3: admission for treatment lasting 6 months.

    Section 136: allows police to take somebody to a place of safety for assessment by a doctor or approved mental healthcare practitioner, lasting 72 hours. **(3)**
4.  As Claire has a condition that is not easily identifiable or does not exhibit prominent physical characteristics, her sense of social rejection may be perceived or 'felt'. An enacted stigma is social rejection that arises from being identified and discredited. **(2)**
5.  Appeal must be applied for in writing to a mental health tribunal within 14 days of detention. **(1)**
6.  Comprehend and retain information about treatment, believing information given, weighing information balance and arriving at a choice. **(3)**

The Mental Health Act is in place to ensure emergency psychiatric care is set to a legislative framework. It covers the assessment, detention and treatment of patients with a psychiatric disorder. Detention against the wishes of the patient without consent is colloquially known as 'sectioning'. For the protection of the patient, a decision to detain somebody for a prolonged period of time is taken by two doctors and an advanced mental health practitioner, usually a social worker. Different sections of the Act refer to different circumstances of detention. The important sections seen commonly in clinical practice are section 2 (admission for assessment), section 3 (admission for treatment), section 5(2) (detention for 72 hours pending full assessment) and section 136 (admission to place of safety by police officers). In order to protect patients, full rights to appeal should be rigorously upheld.

# A⁷

1. BMI < 17.5 kg/m². **(1)**
2. Self-induced vomiting, restrictive diets and increased exercise, use of laxatives/diuretics/appetite suppressants or other weight-loss medication. **(1 mark for each, max 2 marks)**
3. Depression, anxiety, OCD, personality disorder, substance misuse. **(1 mark for each, max 2 marks)**
4. Subfertility, amenorrhoea, anaemia, electrolyte abnormalities (hypokalaemia, hypophosphataemia), hypotension, dental caries from vomiting, brittle and thinning hair, bradycardia, heart failure, osteoporosis, kidney stones. **(1 mark for each, max 2 marks)**
5. Bulimia involves periods of bingeing on food, followed by periods of purging similar to that seen in anorexia. **(1)**
6. Clustering of expertise in one place, supportive group therapy possible, continuous monitoring of patients, capacity for refeeding and monitoring of patients who are severely malnourished. **(1 mark for each, max 2 marks)**
7. Refeeding syndrome. **(1)**

Eating disorders such as anorexia and bulimia nervosa affect many young people of both sexes, although are commoner in females. They involve a pathological fear of weight gain, with distorted cognitions involving weight and body image. This results in severe dieting and weight-loss tactics such as diuretic or laxative abuse, purging and extreme exercise and a BMI < 17.5 kg/m². Low body weight may cause amenorrhoea and other physical effects, such as exhaustion, dizziness, constipation and low blood pressure. More serious problems can occur, such as electrolyte imbalance and malnutrition. Other psychological illness may coexist, such as depression, anxiety, personality disorders and OCD. Management focuses on restoring nutritional balance and body weight, and psychotherapy to address the underlying and maintaining factors of the damaging behaviours. Eating disorder units can involve patients in their own care with group therapy and concentration of specialist services.

# A⁸

1. List each medication taken.

   List any alcohol or illicit drugs also taken.

   When was each medication taken?

   Were they at the same time or were they staggered?

   Psychiatric history.

   Medical history, e.g. liver disease.

   Suicidal intent.

   Immediate triggers to current overdose. **(1 mark for each, max 2 marks)**

2. Activated charcoal, gastric lavage. **(1)**

3. Activated charcoal works by providing a large surface area to absorb a potential poison and stop it from being absorbed by the GI tract; gastric lavage works by removing poisons from the GI tract by an orogastric tube and aspirating contents after inserting large volumes of fluid. **(1)**

4. Patients taking enzyme inducing medications: alcohol, phenytoin, rifampicin, phenobarbitone, etc.

   Patients with reduced hepatic glutathione reserves: HIV-positive, malnourished, anorexic.

   Pre-existing liver disease. **(1 mark for each, max 2 marks)**

5. The toxic metabolite N-acetyl-p-benzoquinone imine (NAPQI) from paracetamol metabolism that causes hepatic damage is detoxified by conjugation with glutathione. In overdose, these glutathione reserves are depleted. NAC provides the liver with enough glutathione to break down NAPQI into a form that can be excreted safely. **(2)**

6. Clotting studies: most important marker for measurement of synthetic liver function.

   LFTs: AST/ALT/bilirubin may also be raised.

   U&Es: acute renal failure is an indication for referral to a specialist unit.

Blood pH: lactic acidosis may be present. **(max 1 mark)**

7. Crisis intervention teams: helpful in instituting positive therapy at the moment of maximum change. They may also reduce admission to psychiatric facilities.

   Social services: especially if she has a poor support network. **(1)**

8. Males 15–30 are more likely to commit completed suicide and are more likely to use a violent method of suicide; females in teenage years and older are more likely to deliberately self-harm or take overdoses. **(2)**

9. Intention of suicide attempt was death, current psychiatric illness, poor social resources, previous suicide attempts, social isolation, male, unemployed, over age 50. **(1 mark for each, max 2 marks)**

10. Specific planning (where, when, how), getting affairs in order, writing a will or a suicide note, having the means to do it, e.g. buying weapons, medications etc. **(1)**

Deliberate self-harm and intentional overdose are common presentations to the emergency department. They may herald a mental illness, such as depression, personality disorder or schizophrenia, or be the result of a patient's intolerable social circumstances, intense pain or avoiding shame. Young adult males are most at risk of a completed suicide and are likely to choose a violent method of death. Often the decision to attempt suicide is an acute event, precipitated by an argument or traumatic event. This situation is where crisis management teams can perform vital interventions. Intentional overdoses may be mixed and require medical admission depending on the substance ingested. Poisons information or Toxbase can help with specific poisons. Worrying features include defined plans for suicide, e.g. suicide note or a will, previous history, professions with access to deadly poisons or weapons. Compulsory admission has to be in the patient's best interests and not just a temporary measure.

# A⁹

1. Legal problems and crime to purchase drugs, abnormal behaviour with signs of intoxication (decreased consciousness, elation, mania), injection marks/abscesses, repeated requests for opioids with other forms of analgesia unacceptable. **(2)**

2. Precontemplative. **(1)**

3. Tailoring of therapeutic intervention to the stage of change the patient is in, to help them move from one stage to another. **(1)**

4. Arbitrary lines are drawn between stages, when in reality patients may go between stages very quickly. The model assumes people make sane and rational choices about their behaviour. **(1)**

5. Cellulitis and abscesses at injection sites, DVT and injection of insoluble debris at injection sites, risk of blood-borne viruses such as hepatitis B, C and HIV, scarred and collapsed veins (making IV access difficult), decreased cognitive function, opportunistic infections from being immunocompromised. **(1 mark for each, max 2 marks)**

6. Methadone: outpatient programmes, requires direct observed dosing and motivated patient.

   Psychological interventions: includes group therapy, motivational enhancement therapy, family and residential programmes.

   Naltrexone rapid detoxification: short-term therapy to be used in conjunction with long-term therapy. Naltrexone competitively blocks opioid receptors. Sedation may be needed for intense withdrawal effects. **(1 mark for each, max 2 marks)**

7. Airway, breathing, circulation, neurological assessment, environmental exposure. **(1)**

8. Naloxone. **(1)**

9. Naloxone has a very short onset and offset of action. Therefore, its effects will wear off quickly (within 5–10 minutes) if given intravenously and opioid toxicity will continue. Intramuscular administration or an infusion should be considered. **(1)**

Substance misuse has a large medical, psychological and societal cost. Individual factors such as gender, personality or family environment interact with cultural and practical factors such as price, availability and legal status to put a person at risk of substance misuse. Harmful behaviours may result in arrest and incarceration, stigmatisation and poverty. Patients may present covertly with requests for narcotic medications or acute severe pain, or overtly in overdose or intoxication. Opiate overdose is potentially fatal and should be treated along standard resuscitation lines and administration of opioid antagonists. Acute withdrawal of opiates can be very distressing for patients and should instigate the commencement of a detoxification programme. Long-term therapy may include psychotherapy, group therapy and inpatient or residential detoxification programmes. There is always a risk of relapse, and long-term follow-up is recommended.

# A¹⁰

1. Abnormal psychological symptoms not attributable to an organic disease or psychosis commonly brought on by stress. **(1)**

2. Tension, agitation, irritability, feeling of impending doom, trembling, palpitations, sense of collapse, hyperventilation (with associated symptoms of tinnitus, tetany, chest pain), headaches, sweating, nausea, hypochondriasis. **(½ a mark for each, max 2 marks)**

3. Panic attack. **(1)**

4. Identifying situations or thoughts that provoke anxiety; recognition that such thoughts cause the anxiety attacks, and aren't correct; therapy alters negative cognitions and teaches coping mechanisms to deal with these situations. **(2)**

5. This is where the therapist evaluates unpleasant effects of various stimuli. The therapist exposes the patient to such situations in increasing levels of unpleasantness, at each increased level calming the patient down using coping mechanisms. The aim is to allow a patient to function in previously unpleasant situations. **(1)**

6. Withdrawal, dependence, tolerance. There are also severe side effects, including drowsiness and reduced consciousness. **(1 mark for each, max 1 mark)**

7. β-blockers, SSRIs, antihistamine. **(1 mark for each, max 2 marks)**

8. Flashbacks, reliving of traumatic event or nightmares of traumatic event, avoidance of stimuli that is associated with trauma, a state of insomnia and anxiety, emotional detachment and decreased responsiveness, hyperactive autonomic nervous system with tachycardia, sweating, increased BP. **(1 mark for each, max 2 marks)**

9. Smoking, alcohol use, avoiding difficult situations. **(max. 1 mark)**

Generalised anxiety disorders are exaggerations of the anxieties that affect us all. They refer to maladaptive psychological symptoms that do not have an organic cause. They can be precipitated by stress. Many physical effects may be present, such as palpitations, chest pain, dyspnoea, and tremor, and may lead the clinician to investigate cardiac abnormalities. Other symptoms include fatigue, insomnia, irritability and obsessions. Cognitive behavioural therapy may be useful in treating the underlying cause of anxiety and may help develop strategies to cope with stressful anxiety-provoking situations. Medications such as benzodiazepines or β-blockers may be used in the short term for acute relief of symptoms. The dangers with medications include drowsiness and rapid development of tolerance and dependence, so these should be used with care.

# Paediatrics

## A¹

1. Fever, tachycardia, tachypnoea, wheeze, apnoea, respiratory distress – intercostal, subcostal and supraclavicular recession, tracheal tug, nasal flaring, cyanosis crepitations. (½ **a mark each, max 2)**
2. Respiratory syncytial virus. **(1)**
3. Nasopharyngeal aspiration. **(1)**
4. Rib recession, apnoea, > 50 breaths per minute, dehydration, poor feeding, patient or parental exhaustion. (½ **a mark for each, max 3)**
5. Oxygen, NG feeding. **(2)**
6. Hyperinflation. **(1)**

Acute bronchiolitis is a lower respiratory infection that affects infants, usually under 2 years in age. Respiratory syncytial virus is the usual causative virus and can be confirmed by taking a nasopharyngeal aspirate. Treatment is supportive, the reasons for hospital admission are listed. Ensuring adequate oxygenation, nutrition and hydration are key. Ventilation may be needed in the severely ill.

## A²

1. Barking cough, sounding like a seal's bark. **(1)**
2. Hoarseness, stridor. **(2)**
3. Epiglotitis, foreign body, anaphylaxis. **(2)**
4. Parainfluenza virus, respiratory syncytial virus, influenza, measles, adenovirus. **(1 mark for each, max 2 marks)**
5. Steroids – usually dexamethasone. **(1)**
6. Nebulised adrenaline. **(1)**
7. Respiratory distress (rib recession, tracheal tug, nasal flaring), restlessness, cyanosis, rising pulse, rising respiratory rate, lethargy. (½ **a mark each, max 2 marks)**

Croup (acute laryngotracheobronchitis) is an upper respiratory tract infection usually caused by parainfluenza virus. The virus causes subglottic oedema and inflammation, which causes a 'barking' cough, hoarseness and stridor. Dexamethasone is usually given as a one-off treatment and parents are told what to watch out for. In severe disease, nebulised adrenaline is also given, and if no response the patient will be taken to intensive care.

## A³

1. 2–8 weeks. **(1)**
2. The stenosis causes an obstruction too high for bile to be present in the vomit. **(2)**
3. 'Projectile'. **(1)**
4. Lateral border of the rectus in the right upper quadrant. **(1)**
5. Metabolic alkalosis. **(1)**
6. Cardia, fundus, body, pylorus. **(½ a mark for each, max 2 marks)**
7. Hypokalaemia, hypochloraemia. **(2)**

Congenital hypertrophic pyloric stenosis usually presents at 2–8 weeks of age. Vomiting is typically after feeding, at usually large volumes and 'projectile' in nature. Bile is not in the vomit as the obstruction is too high. A hypokalaemic, hypochloraemic metabolic alkalosis develops. If the presentation is early, the enlarged pylorus may not be felt. In this case, an ultrasound can be used. Management is surgical.

## A⁴

1. Male. **(1)**
2. 10–17 years. **(1)**
3. Obesity, local trauma, hormone deficiencies (hypothyroidism, hypopituitarism, growth hormone deficiency), chemotherapy, radiotherapy. **(1 mark for each, max 2 marks)**
4. Hyaline cartilage. **(1)**
5. Limp on walking, external rotation of limb, hip motion is limited (flexion, abduction and medial rotation). **(1 mark for each, max 2 marks)**
6. Perthes' disease, acute transient synovitis (irritable hip), septic arthritis, osteomyelitis, hip fracture. **(1 mark for each, max 3 marks)**

A slipped upper femoral epiphysis tends to occur in males in the age range of 10–17 years. It presents with hip or knee pain, causing a limp. It often cannot be seen on AP radiograph, so lateral radiographs need to be taken. Avascular necrosis of the femoral head or malunion can occur if untreated. Analgesia, avoiding moving the leg and an orthopaedic review should be sought. Definitive treatment includes a corrective osteotomy or with screws.

# A5

1. Yellowing of the skin and sclera **(1)** due to raised levels of bilirubin in the circulation. **(1)**
2. Rhesus haemolytic disease, ABO incompatibility, hereditary spherocytosis, G6PD deficiency, haematomas, toxoplasmosis, syphilis, rubella, cytomegalovirus, herpes, hepatitis. **(2)**
3. FBC, blood groups, direct Coombs' test, blood film, TORCH screen, urine-reducing substances, urine dipstick/microscopy. **(2)**
4. Biliary atresia. **(1)**
5. Kernicterus. **(1)**
6. Phototherapy, exchange transfusion. **(2)**

Neonatal jaundice is a very common presentation to paediatricians. It is due to raised levels of bilirubin in the circulation causing yellowing of the skin and sclera. A raised level of unconjugated jaundice may be due to a physiological or pathological cause and has the potential to be toxic due to its ability to cross the blood-brain barrier. A raised level of conjugated bilirubin is always due to a pathological cause, but is not toxic as it cannot cross the blood-brain barrier. Jaundice within the first 24 hours of life is always abnormal, and the causes and investigations are discussed above. Jaundice present after 14 days in term babies and 21 days in premature babies is known as prolonged jaundice. Causes include breastfeeding, infections (UTI, TORCH), endocrine abnormalities (hypothyroidism, hypopituitarism), metabolic abnormalities (cystic fibrosis, galactosaemia, alpha-1-antitrypsin deficiency) and biliary atresia. Physiological jaundice typically occurs between 2 and 14 days and is due to increased erythrocyte breakdown and hepatic immaturity. Babies presenting with jaundice should have their total bilirubin level measured as soon as possible and their level plotted on the admitting hospital's protocol. If the level of jaundice requires treatment, options include phototherapy and exchange transfusion. The risk of untreated raised unconjugated bilirubin is kernicterus, which is when unconjugated bilirubin crosses the blood-brain barrier and forms deposits in the basal ganglia and brainstem, giving rise to neurological complications.

# A⁶

1. Echocardiography. **(1)**
2. Left-to-right shunting of blood. **(1)**
3. Atrial septal defect, ventral septal defect, patent ductus arteriosus, coarctation of the aorta, pulmonary stenosis, aortic stenosis. **(2)**
4. Right-to-left shunting of blood. **(1)**
5. Fallot's tetralogy, transposition of the great arteries, tricuspid atresia, pulmonary atresia, hypoplastic left heart, truncus arteriosus, total anomalous pulmonary venous return. **(2)**
6. Poor feeding, dypnoea, tachycardia, weak pulse, cold peripheries, hepatomegaly, engorged neck veins, sweating, gallop rhythm (third heart sound). **(2)**
7. When a left-to-right shunt leads to pulmonary hypertension and shunt reversal, therefore turning an acyanotic heart defect into a cyanotic heart defect. **(1)**

Congenital heart disease encompasses a variety of heart abnormalities, ranging from small asymptomatic defects to more severe life-threatening forms. Many are diagnosed on antenatal scans, but those not picked up by these scans may present with murmurs on screening, difficulty feeding, breathlessness, cyanosis or tachycardia. It is important to note that some defects such as ventricular septal defects may not present until the ductus arteriosus closes when the pulmonary vascular resistance changes. Some defects do not require any management, but others may require such interventions as balloon valvulotomy, surgical correction or heart transplant.

# A⁷

1. Maternal diabetes, Caesarean sections, second twins, males, hypothermia, perinatal asphyxia, family history of IRDS. **(2)**
2. Surfactant. **(1)**
3. Type II pneumocytes. **(1)**
4. Steroids – dexamethasone/betamethasone. **(1)**
5. Tachypnoea, cyanosis, grunting, nasal flaring, recession. **(2)**
6. Diffuse granular shadowing/ground-glass shadowing. **(1)**

7.  Choose an appropriate setting, ensure there are no interruptions, use a warning shot, determine the depth of information the person/people being informed wish to know, encourage them to express their emotions, summarise, make a follow-up plan. **(2)**

IRDS is the main cause of death in premature babies. It is due to insufficient surfactant in the lungs. Prior to birth, steroids may be used to prevent IRDS. Following birth, the treatment is via intubation and administration of surfactant via the endotracheal tube.

# A⁸

1.  Six months to 5 years old. **(1)**
2.  Focal signs, duration of more than 15 minutes, recurrence within 24 hours, incomplete recovery within 1 hour. **(2)**
3.  FBC, blood culture, U&Es, glucose, chest X-ray, urine dipstick and MSU, throat swab, lumbar puncture. **(3)**
4.  Benzodiazepines. **(1)**
5.  What febrile convulsions are, how to manage pyrexia at home, first aid for seizures, when to call an ambulance. **(3)**

Febrile convulsions occur as temperatures rise rapidly in febrile illnesses. Common causes include tonsillitis, otitis media and gastroenteritis. More serious causes which must be excluded are meningitis, urinary tract infections and lower respiratory tract infections. Initial management is via putting the patient in the recovery position ABCDE approach. If the seizure continues for more than 5 minutes, a benzodiazepine should be administered either IV, buccal or PR. An antipyretic should be given if feasible. Once the patient is ready for discharge, parental education is vital. It is important to tell them that this isn't epilepsy and that only a very small percentage of children who have febrile convulsions go on to develop epilepsy. They should be counselled on how to manage pyrexia, such as removing excess clothing, giving antipyretics and plenty of fluid. Parents should be counselled on how to perform first aid, and for children who have recurrent febrile convulsions, how to administer buccal midazolam or PR diazepam.

# A⁹

1. A chronic disorder of movement and posture **(1)** due to non-progressive brain abnormalities **(1)** occurring before the brain is fully developed.
2. Spastic, athetoid, ataxic, mixed. **(2)**
3. Delayed milestones, failure to thrive, epilepsy, urinary incontinence, constipation, drooling, sleep disturbance, contractures. **(2)**
4. Nurses, physiotherapists, occupational therapists, speech and language therapists, recreational therapists, orthoses experts. **(2)**
5. Baclofen, diazepam, dantrolene. **(2)**

Cerebral palsy will often present with a delay in achieving milestones, in particular a delay in walking, which is usually achieved by the age of 14 months. Prenatal causes include infection, teratogens and hypoxia. Birth trauma is a cause of cerebral palsy, but is less common than prenatal factors. Other causes include hypoglycaemia, hyperbilirubinaemia and intraventricular haemorrhage. The aim of management in children with cerebral palsy is to ensure a good quality of life and integration into society. This is achieved using a multidisciplinary team approach. It is also important to ensure the well-being of carers is not overlooked.

# A¹⁰

1. Males. **(1)**
2. Sausage-shaped abdominal mass. **(1)**
3. One segment of bowel telescopes into a distal segment of bowel, causing obstruction. **(1)**
4. Right lower quadrant opacity, dilated gas-filled proximal bowel with absence of gas distally, multiple fluid levels, perforation. **(2)**
5. FBC, U&E, ultrasound scan, bowel enema (barium/water-soluble/air), CT scan, MRI scan. **(2)**
6. Reduction by enema. **(1)**
7. Perforation, peritonitis, prolonged history, failed enema, high likelihood of pathological cause. **(1 mark for each, max 2 marks)**

Intussusception occurs when part of the bowel telescopes into another part, causing obstruction. It most commonly occurs in the ileocaecal region. This may occur spontaneously or may be due to such pathology as Meckel's diverticulum, Peutz-Jeghers syndrome or Henoch–Schönlein purpura. Paroxysms of colicky abdominal pain occur, during which patients may be shocked. However, between paroxysms patients may appear well. Early management includes resuscitation by a 'drip and suck' technique via a nasogastric tube, and IV fluids. Reduction via enema may avoid the need for surgery. Prognosis is excellent with early treatment, but if left untreated intussusception may be fatal.

# Practice paper

**Q1** A 33-year-old lady is admitted with severe, sharp central chest pain that is worse when lying down, moving and deep inspiration. She is sat on the edge of the bed and refusing to lie down, as sitting forward relieves the pain slightly. She is given analgesia, becomes more compliant with your examination and you hear a pericardial rub. You request a number of investigations, including an ECG.

1. What is the most likely diagnosis? **(1)**
2. Give other causes of this condition. **(3)**
3. What abnormality may be seen on the ECG of a patient with the above diagnosis? **(1)**

Cardiac tamponade is a potential complication of this condition. Beck's triad may be found on examination of this patient.

4. What is cardiac tamponade? **(1)**
5. How is cardiac tamponade managed? **(1)**
6. What is Beck's triad? **(3)**

**Q2** A 32-year-old man is taken to A&E with sudden onset of right-sided, pleuritic chest pain. Investigations reveal a right-sided pneumothorax. It is not believed to be under tension.

1. Give two signs you may expect to find on examination of his chest. **(2)**
2. If this was a tension pneumothorax, what additional sign may you find? **(1)**
3. Indicate how you would manage a suspected tension pneumothorax, including anatomical landmarks. **(2)**
4. Give three possible causes of pneumothorax. **(3)**
5. The pneumothorax is estimated to represent 15% of the radiographic volume. Approximately how long will this take to reabsorb? **(1)**
6. He is due to fly to Spain in 6 days. What advice would you give him regarding air travel? **(1)**

**Q3** A 36-year-old lady is seen in the renal clinic. Her GP had arranged a USS due to ongoing loin pain, which has revealed polycstic kidneys. She has two sisters, aged 32 and 30, who are both fit and well. Her father is also in good health, but her mother died suddenly aged 42 from 'a bleed on the brain'.

1. What is the mode of inheritance of polycystic kidney disease? **(1)**
2. Name the gene commonly responsible for this form of polycystic kidneys. **(1)**
3. How do you suspect her mother died and why? **(2)**
4. Give two signs you may find on examination. **(2)**
5. Give three other possible complications of polycystic kidneys other than a 'bleed on the brain'. **(3)**
6. What advice would you give her regarding her family? **(1)**

**Q4** A 76-year-old lady visits her GP. She has had a headache that has been troubling her for 2–3 days, for which she has been taking paracetamol. She would not normally have troubled her GP, but was alarmed the previous night when she temporarily lost vision in her right eye, describing it as 'a curtain being closed'. On examination, she is tender over the right temple. Her past medical history includes hypertension and polymyalgia rheumatica, for which she is currently taking 4 mg prednisolone daily.

1. What is the most likely diagnosis? **(1)**
2. What is the main concern if this condition is not treated promptly? **(1)**
3. What treatment should be initiated immediately? **(1)**
4. Blood tests arranged by the GP reveal a raised ESR (95 mm/h). What investigation would you request to confirm the diagnosis? **(1)**
5. What is the name given to her visual symptoms? **(1)**
6. Give five side effects of steroids. **(5)**

Q5 A 63-year-old lady with severe COPD comes to see you in the GP practice, complaining of weight gain around her abdomen (despite no change to her diet) and feeling low in mood. For her COPD, she is taking salbutamol, ipratropium, oral steroids and home oxygen. On examination, you notice thinning of her skin and also a moon-face appearance.

1. What is the syndrome called which explains her history and examination findings? What do you think the cause is in this lady's case? **(2)**
2. Name two other signs you might find on examination of this lady. **(2)**

Another patient comes to see you with similar symptoms and examination findings as well as having a tanned appearance despite no excess sun exposure. However, this patient has no past medical history and no drug history.

3. What is Cushing's disease? **(1)**
4. Suggest two initial investigations you would like to perform. **(2)**
5. What imaging studies would you request for any Cushingoid patient? **(2)**
6. How do you explain her tanned appearance? **(1)**

**Q6** Gladys is a 74-year-old lady admitted to one of the medical wards for the elderly, with a UTI causing her to be confused. She is started on antibiotics. She is usually fit and well with no confusion. She is taking warfarin for a DVT diagnosed 4 months ago.

1. Name four risk factors for developing a deep vein thrombosis. **(2)**
2. What is the target INR range for the treatment of idiopathic venous thromboembolism? **(1)**
3. If this was her first DVT with no cause found, how long would she have to be treated with warfarin for? **(1)**

Whilst in hospital, she has a fall during the night, causing a fracture of her neck of femur. The orthopaedic consultant wants her to be anticoagulated prior to operating on her.

4. Name three treatment options to reduce Gladys' INR. **(3)**
5. What other form of treatment should be given to the patient to stop her from developing further clots prior to her surgery? **(2)**

Her surgery goes well; however, whilst recovering in hospital she goes on to suffer from a further DVT which embolises to the lungs.

6. How long will Gladys have to remain on warfarin for now? **(1)**

**Q7** Lee, aged 34, presents to the emergency department with sudden onset severe epigastric pain and vomiting.

1. List four causes of acute epigastric pain. **(2)**
2. Name a radiological investigation you would use in this case in the emergency department. **(1)**
3. Lee's amylase comes back as 1340. List three causes of pancreatitis. **(3)**
4. Lee's Glasgow score is 3. What implication does this have on his management? **(1)**
5. List two criteria to calculate a Glasgow score. **(1)**
6. How would you treat pancreatitis initially? **(2)**
7. Why would a USS abdomen be useful in this case? **(1)**
8. On the post-take ward round the next morning, your consultant notices some bruising on the patient's flank. What is the eponym for this sign and what does it represent? **(2)**
9. Name two complications of acute pancreatitis. **(2)**

8 A 45-year-old woman is seen in the neurology outpatients' clinic due to drooping of her eyelids and double vision. A diagnosis of myasthenia gravis is suspected.

1. Myasthenia gravis is an autoimmune condition. What aspect of the neuromuscular junction do the autoantibodies produced act on? **(1)**
2. Give two other autoimmune conditions associated with myasthenia gravis. **(2)**
3. Which tumour is myasthenia gravis associated with? **(1)**
4. What is the defining feature about the muscle weakness? **(1)**
5. Give two investigations that may be performed to aid in diagnosis. **(2)**
6. Give two treatment options. **(2)**
7. What life-threatening complication may occur in a patient with myasthenia gravis? **(1)**

9 A 60-year-old man attends your GP clinic with dizziness. On further questioning, it is found that he has lost 2 stone over the last few months and feels tired all the time. He is a little overweight and enjoys his food and wine. He has hypertension and hypercholesterolaemia. You suspect colon cancer.

1. How does the presentation of cancer in the large bowel change with location? Compare the right and left sides. **(2)**
2. How else can bowel cancers present acutely? **(2)**
3. Give four predisposing factors for bowel cancer. **(2)**
4. What investigations should be performed? Name two. **(2)**
5. How is colon cancer classically staged? **(1)**
6. What is the commonest histological diagnosis for colorectal cancer? **(1)**

**Q10** An 18-year-old girl presents to her GP with a swelling in her neck. On examination, there is a midline mass which moves upwards on protrusion of the tongue.
1. What is the likely diagnosis? **(1)**
2. Give two other causes of a midline mass. **(2)**
3. Using embryology, explain how this condition arises. **(2)**
4. What are two possible complications of the condition. **(2)**
5. Give two investigations which may be performed. **(2)**
6. What is the treatment for this condition? **(1)**

**Q11** A midwife comes to you seeking your attention urgently on the delivery suite. It is regarding a 36-year-old lady who has only 20 minutes ago delivered twins; she is a para 8, and delivery of the second twin took longer than expected. She is bleeding heavily from her genital tract. You estimate she has lost over 1 L of blood.
1. What is the definition of primary post-partum haemorrhage (PPH)? **(1)**
2. Name four risk factors for post-partum haemorrhage. **(2)**
3. What are the four main causes of post-partum haemorrhage, and which of these account for the most cases of post-partum haemorrhage? **(3)**
4. What is the most likely cause in this patient? **(1)**
5. What would be your initial management in this patient? **(1)**
6. Name two drugs that could be administered to specifically treat this patient's problems. **(2)**

**Q12** Barbara, aged 62, has come to see you as she has symptoms of urine leak, and feeling of a mass in her vagina.

1. How is female continence maintained? **(1)**
2. Name a risk factor for vaginal prolapse. **(1)**
3. Define the following terms: cystocoele, rectocoele and stress incontinence. **(3)**
4. Name two common medical problems that will make urine incontinence worse. **(1)**
5. What investigation should you send Barbara for, to assess her incontinence? **(1)**
6. Investigations show Barbara has predominantly urge incontinence. What lifestyle changes can help in urge incontinence? **(2)**
7. What medical treatments can be used in urge incontinence? **(1)**

**Q13** A 22-year-old man has had severe asthma since childhood, requiring numerous hospital admissions. He presents via A&E short of breath, coughing and complaining his chest feels tight. His symptoms have been getting progressively worse over the last 2 days and he has been using his 'reliever' every couple of hours, but it is no longer helping. Venous blood tests taken on admission are all within normal limits. His regular medications are listed below:

- salbutamol CFC-free 100 mcg, actuation 2 puffs BD
- seretide 250 evohaler (fluticasone 250 mcg/salmeterol 25 mcg), 2 puffs twice daily.

1. Give three features of acute severe asthma. **(3)**
2. Give two further investigations you would request. **(2)**
3. Name two drugs, other than those he is currently taking, that may be used to manage acute exacerbations of asthma. **(2)**
4. Using the BTS guidelines, name one drug that may be appropriately added to his asthma regimen at this stage. **(1)**
5. He is admitted for 4 days and recovers well. Prior to discharge, give two checks you can make or advice you can give to reduce the risk of future exacerbations. **(2)**

**Q14** A 6-year-old boy with known cystic fibrosis is seen in your GP clinic. His mother is concerned that he has lost weight.

1. What proportion of Caucasians carry one allele for cystic fibrosis? **(1)**
2. Name two different tests for diagnosing cystic fibrosis. **(2)**
3. Name two potential pulmonary complications from cystic fibrosis. **(2)**
4. What is the likely cause for the malnutrition? **(1)**
5. Give two other gastrointestinal complications related to cystic fibrosis. **(2)**
6. What is steatorrhoea? **(1)**
7. What are the fat-soluble vitamins? **(2)**

**Q15** A 22-year-old male is brought into the resuscitation department of A&E after sustaining major thermal burns. They occurred due to a house fire in an enclosed space. He is assessed and managed initially using the ABCDE approach.

1. Give two modalities of sustaining burns other than thermal injuries. **(2)**
2. Why is it essential to assess this patient's airway as early as possible? **(1)**
3. Give one method of assessing the body surface area affected by burns. **(1)**
4. List two differences between superficial burns and full-thickness burns on examination. **(2)**
5. What is the Parkland formula for calculating the volume of intravenous Hartmann's solution to be given over 24 hours? **(1)**
6. How should the administration of the calculated fluid be divided over the 24-hour period? **(1)**
7. What are the two commonest causes of death in burns patients? **(2)**

# Answers

## A¹

1. Acute pericarditis. **(1)**
2. Viruses (e.g. coxsachievirus, influenza, HIV), bacteria (e.g. *Staphylococcus*, *Streptococcus*, TB), fungi (e.g. histoplasmosis), post-MI (Dressler's syndrome), malignancy, uraemia, radiation, trauma, autoimmune (rheumatoid arthritis, SLE, systemic sclerosis), drugs (hydralazine, procainamide, isoniazid). **(1 mark for each, max 3 marks)**
3. Saddle-shaped ST-segment elevation. **(1)**
4. Accumulation of pericardial fluid causing increased pericardial pressure which compromises ventricular filling, resulting in a reduced cardiac output. **(1)**
5. Pericardiocentesis. **(1)**
6. Falling blood pressure, rising JVP, muffled heart sounds. **(1 mark for each, max 3 marks)**

The aetiology of acute pericarditis is usually viral or autoimmune. Patients typically present with severe chest pain that is worse on lying down. Saddle-shaped ST elevation is the classical ECG finding, but many patients will have a normal ECG. NSAIDs are often the most effective form of analgesia in these patients. If an autoimmune cause is found, steroids and immunosuppressants may be necessary. A pericardial effusion is a possible complication of pericarditis, and if the effusion is large enough to compromise cardiac filling, this is known as cardiac tamponade. Beck's triad is typically seen on examination. Management of this is pericardiocentesis. This involves insertion of a needle into the pericardial sac, and aspiration of fluid. Complications of this procedure include myocardial damage, damage to the coronary arteries, arrhythmias and pneumothorax.

# A²

1. Reduced chest expansion on the affected side, hyperresonant percussion note on the affected side, diminished breath sounds on the affected side. **(1 mark for each, max 2 marks)**

2. Tracheal deviation away from the affected side. **(1)**

3. Insertion of wide-bore cannula into second intercostal space, mid-clavicular line on the affected side **(1 mark for management, 1 mark for landmarks, max 2 marks)**

4. Idiopathic, asthma, COPD, trauma, lung cancer, pneumonia, lung abscess, TB, sarcoidosis, barotrauma, cystic fibrosis, other connective tissue disorders (e.g. Marfan's syndrome, Ehlers–Danlos syndrome), iatrogenic (e.g. mechanical ventilation, CVP line insertion). **(1 mark for each, max 3 marks)**

5. 12 days (1.25% per day). **(1)**

6. Air travel should be avoided until full resolution confirmed on chest X-ray, so not safe to fly. **(1)**

The term 'pneumothorax' refers to the presence of air within the pleural space. A small pneumothorax may cause no symptoms. Others may present with pleuritic chest pain and shortness of breath. Spontaneous pneumothoraces occur most commonly in young men following the rupture of a pleural bleb. Other causes of pneumothorax include asthma, COPD, TB and connective tissue disorders, such as Marfan's syndrome or Ehlers–Danlos syndrome. Management options include aspiration of the pneumothorax or insertion of a chest drain. A tension pneumothorax is a medical emergency. A one-way valve forms, allowing air to be drawn into the pleura but does not allow it to be expelled. This causes increased pressure and forces the mediastinum towards the contralateral hemithorax, compressing the great veins. This is most commonly seen in patients receiving positive pressure ventilation, and causes worsening respiratory distress, hypotension, distended neck veins and tracheal deviation away from the affected side, as well as the other signs associated with a pneumothorax. Treatment is to convert the pneumothorax to an open pneumothorax immediately with needle thoracocentesis. It is important to remember that a pneumothorax may also occur following trauma, such as a road traffic accident. These cases should be managed by inserting a chest drain.

# A³

1. Autosomal dominant. **(1)**
2. *PKD1.* **(1)**
3. Subarachnoid haemorrhage, increased incidence of berry aneurysms in those with polycystic kidneys. **(1 mark for cause, 1 mark for risk, max 2 marks)**
4. Hypertension, palpable kidneys (large, irregular). hepatomegaly, mitral valve prolapse (mid-systolic click and/or late systolic murmur). **(1 mark for each, max 2 marks)**
5. Chronic renal failure, hypertension, renal calculi, cyst infection, chronic pain, hepatic cysts, haematuria. **(1 mark for each, max 3 marks)**
6. First-degree relatives should be screened for the presence of polycystic kidneys. **(1)**

Most cases of polycystic kidney disease are due to the autosomal dominant form. It is characterised by numerous renal cysts. Local complications include pain, bleeding into cysts, infected cysts and renal calculi. Complications elsewhere include the development of hepatic cysts, mitral valve prolapse and berry aneurysms, which may rupture, causing subarachnoid haemorrhage. Progressive renal failure often develops at a rate faster than other primary renal conditions, and many require some form of renal replacement therapy. First-degree relatives should be screened due to its autosomal dominant inheritance.

# A⁴

1. Temporal/giant cell arteritis. **(1)**
2. Irreversible blindness. **(1)**
3. High-dose steroids. **(1)**
4. Temporal artery biopsy. **(1)**
5. Amaurosis fugax. **(1)**
6. Osteoporosis, hypertension, hyperglycaemia/DM, altered fat distribution (moon face, buffalo hump, central obesity), cataracts, bruising, striae, skin thinning, immunosuppression, muscle wasting, psychosis, avascular necrosis of the femoral head. **(1 mark for each, max 5 marks)**

Temporal arteritis often presents with headache and temporal artery tenderness. Other symptoms may include jaw claudication and visual disturbance. The main concern is irreversible blindness, which may occur in both eyes, and therefore requires a high index of suspicion. If temporal arteritis is suspected, an ESR should be requested, the patient should be started on steroids and a temporal artery biopsy should be performed within the next few days. This often confirms the diagnosis, but skip lesions may be seen and a negative biopsy does not rule it out. Most cases settle with steroids within 2 years. There is an association with polymyalgia rheumatica in 25% of cases.

# A5

1. Cushing's syndrome, iatrogenic secondary to the steroids she is taking for her COPD. **(1 mark for each)**
2. Bruising, purple striae on abdomen, buffalo hump, high blood pressure, proximal myopathy. **(1 mark for each, max 2 marks)**
3. Hypersecretion of ACTH from a pituitary adenoma. **(1)**
4. 24-h urinary cortisol, dexamethasone depression test, midnight cortisol. **(1 mark for each, max 2 marks)**
5. MRI pituitary, CT abdomen, CXR. **(1 mark for each, max 2 marks)**
6. ACTH has a stimulatory effect on melanocytes as there is affinity for the MSH receptor. **(1)**

Cushing's syndrome is not Cushing's disease. The commonest cause of Cushing's syndrome is steroid therapy. If the patient is not on steroid therapy, then other causes must be looked for with the use of biochemical tests and imaging. In the dexamethasone suppression test, serum cortisol measurements are taken after giving high doses of steroid. In a normal patient, there is negative feedback which causes decreased production of ACTH and therefore decreased serum cortisol. In Cushing's syndrome and Cushing's disease, there is failure to suppress cortisol production.

# A6

1. Obesity, malignancy, acute inflammation, reduced mobility, surgery, oestrogen therapy, pregnancy, past history, clotting disorders, long-haul air travel, dehydration. **(2)**
2. 2–3. **(1)**
3. Six months. **(1)**

4. Fresh frozen plasma, vitamin K, prothrombin complex (beriplex or octoplex). **(3)**
5. Low molecular weight heparin, compression stockings. **(2)**
6. Lifelong. **(1)**

There are multiple risk factors for DVT. When patients come into hospital, they are risk-assessed for thromboprophylaxis, so nearly all patients receive low-dose low molecular weight heparin (LMWH) once daily as inpatients. If venous thromboembolism does develop, then therapeutic doses of LMWH (e.g. enoxaparin 1.5 mg/kg) are given alongside warfarin until the INR is in therapeutic range. LMWH acts by inhibiting factor Xa. Warfarin works by inhibiting the synthesis of clotting factors X, IX, VII and II. Vitamin K can be used to reverse the INR; however, it takes a long time to act (6–12 hours) and can cause a longer time to reanticoagulate patients after, depending on the dose of vitamin K given. Fresh frozen plasma and prothrombin complexes act a lot more quickly. If patients suffer with repeat VTE episodes, then they are anticoagulated permanently.

# A⁷

1. Acute pancreatitis, gastritis, myocardial infarction, abdominal aortic aneurysm, perforated peptic ulcer, cholecystitis. **(½ a mark for each, max 2 marks)**
2. Erect chest X-ray to look for pneumoperitoneum suggestive of perforation. **(1)**
3. Gallstones, alcohol, trauma, hyperlipidaemia, post-ERCP, post-surgery, medications (NSAIDS, steroids, azathioprine, isoniazid), mumps, CMV, scorpion venom, idiopathic. **(1 mark for each, max 3 marks)**
4. A Glasgow score of 3 or higher is suggestive of severe pancreatitis with a high chance of developing SIRS/multi-organ dysfunction. The implication for management is that Lee should be managed in HDU/ITU. **(1)**
5. Modified Glasgow Score: 
   $pO_2 < 10\,kPa$
   Age > 55 years
   White cell count $> 15\,000 \times 10^9$
   Corrected calcium < 2 mmol/L
   Urea > 7 mmol/L
   ALT > 100 IU/L

Albumin < 35 g/L

Glucose > 7 mmol/L

**(½ a mark for each, max 1 mark)**

6. Treatment is initially supportive with IV fluid resuscitation and monitoring fluid balance with urinary catheterisation. Treat pain with analgesia and vomiting with anti-emetics. Some centres use early enteral feeding and IV antibiotics in severe cases. Definitive treatment depends on the cause, e.g. gallstones or alcohol.
   **(1 mark for each, max 2 marks)**

7. Ultrasound abdomen can be used to assess for presence of gallstones in the gallbladder, common bile duct or pancreatic duct.
   **(1)**

8. Grey Turner's sign is bruising along the flanks and is seen in haemorrhagic pancreatitis. It represents retroperitoneal and intra-abdominal bleeding where altered blood tracks subcutaneously. Similar bruising around the umbilicus is known as Cullen's sign.
   **(2)**

9. Sepsis from bacterial translocation, acute respiratory distress syndrome, stress peptic ulceration, multi-organ dysfunction, pancreatic pseudocyst, infected pancreatic necrosis, chronic pancreatitis, diabetes mellitus. **(1 mark for each, max 2 marks)**

Acute pancreatitis is a common emergency presentation and requires swift treatment as it has a not-insignificant mortality. It is an inflammatory process where pro-inflammatory cytokines (TNF-alpha, IL-2, IL-6) and pancreatic digestive enzymes (trypsin, lipase, amylase) are released in response to pancreatic insult. The inflammatory response may be sufficient for multi-organ dysfunction or SIRS. The two commonest causes in the UK are gallstones and alcohol abuse, with many other much rarer causes listed above. Symptoms include severe epigastric and back pain with nausea and vomiting, fever, tachycardia and hypotension. Management is supportive, with aggressive fluid replacement requiring catheterisation and sometimes central venous pressure monitoring. Severe cases may require ITU admission for renal replacement therapy, cardiovascular and ventilatory support. CT scanning can identify collections, necrosis or haemorrhage and can be used to guide drainage of such collections. In cases where gallstones are the cause, urgent ERCP can remove stones, and the gallbladder should be removed when the patient is stable.

## A8

1. Nicotinic acetylcholine receptors at the post-synaptic neuromuscular junction. (1)
2. Graves' disease, Hashimoto's thyroiditis, rheumatoid arthritis, SLE, diabetes mellitus type 1, pernicious anaemia. (2)
3. Thymoma. (1)
4. Fatigability – the weakness is worse on exercise and better with rest. (1)
5. Blood tests (antiacetylcholine receptor antibody, anti-MuSK antibodies, antistriated muscle antibody), Tensilon test, neurophysiology studies, muscle biopsy, CT/MRI to detect thymoma. (1 mark for each, max 2 marks)
6. Acetylcholinesterase inhibitors (e.g. neostigmine, pyridostigmine), immunosuppression (e.g. prednisolone, azathioprine, ciclosporin), plasmapheresis, intravenous immunoglobulins, thymectomy. (2)
7. Acute respiratory failure due to weakness of the muscles of ventilation. (1)

Myasthenia gravis is an autoimmune condition due to antibodies targeted against the nicotinic acetylcholine receptors on the post-synaptic neuromuscular junction. It is associated with thymomas and a number of autoimmune conditions. The clinical presentation of myasthenia gravis is of muscular weakness which is characterised by fatigability (i.e. worsens on exercise). The extraocular muscles are often the first muscle group affected, followed by bulbar, facial and proximal muscle groups. The Tensilon test is an investigation used to aid in diagnosis. This involves administering a short-acting acetylcholinesterase inhibitor (edrophonium) to the patient and watching for an improvement in the muscle weakness. However, due to the risk of increased vagal tone producing bradycardia, the test should only be performed where resuscitation facilities and atropine are to hand. Thymectomy is indicated in patients with a thymoma but may also benefit patients without one, so is often considered in younger patients and when acetylcholinesterase inhibitors are ineffective.

# A⁹

1. Right-sided – weight loss, anaemia, abdominal pain; left-sided – bleeding/mucus per rectum, tenesmus, altered bowel habit. **(1 mark for right-sided symptoms, 1 for left-sided, max 2 marks)**
2. Perforation, obstruction, haemorrhage, fistula. **(2)**
3. Family history, inflammatory bowel disease, slow transit time, adenomatous polyposis, hereditary non-polyposis colon cancer. **(1 mark for each, max 2 marks)**
4. FBC, faecal, colonoscopy, CT colonoscopy, barium enema, barium follow-through, capsule endoscopy. **(1)**
5. Duke's classification. **(1)**
6. Adenocarcinoma. **(1)**

Duke's classification is used for the staging of colorectal cancer. Stage A is confined beneath muscularis mucosae, Stage B extends through the muscularis mucosae, Stage C is involved in regional lymph nodes and Stage D has distant metastases. Colonoscopy is the most accurate test, as it visualises the entire colon and allows for biopsy. It is used as an investigation or as surveillance in those with a significant family or personal history, adenoma or inflammatory bowel disease.

# A¹⁰

1. Thyroglossal cyst. **(1)**
2. Dermoid cyst, thyroid mass, thymus mass, chondroma. **(2)**
3. The thyroid gland begins its development at the foramen caecum (junction between anterior 2/3 and posterior 1/3 of the tongue), and then migrates to the base of the neck but remains connected to the tongue by the thyroglossal duct. Cysts can arise anywhere along this pathway. **(2)**
4. Malignancy, infection, airway compromise, dysphagia. **(2)**
5. TFTs, USS, CT scan, thyroid scan (using radioactive iodine/technetium). **(2)**
6. Surgical excision. **(1)**

Thyroglossal cysts are fluctuant midline swellings which arise anywhere along the thyroglossal duct. Possible complications include malignancy, infection and, if the cysts grow large enough, airway compromise and dysphagia. Prior to surgery to excise the cysts, TFTs and thyroid scans should be performed to demonstrate normal thyroid position and function prior to potentially removing thyroid tissue which may be present in the cyst.

# A¹¹

1. > 500 ml blood loss from genital tract within 24 hours of delivery. **(1)**
2. Prolonged labour, grand multiparity, multiple gestation, polyhydramnios, retained placenta, coagulation problems, instrumental delivery, previous Caesarean section, previous PPH. **(2)**
3. The four Ts (tone, tissue, thrombin, trauma): uterine atony, accounts for up to 90% of cases; retained tissue; coagulation defects; trauma. **(3)**
4. Uterine atony. **(1)**
5. Check airway, breathing and circulation and correct abnormalities at each stage. **(1)**
6. Ergometrine, oxytocin, carboprost/haemabate. **(2)**

Post-partum haemorrhage can in some cases be life-threatening. In cases with such risk factors as the lady in the scenario above, the patient should be admitted to the delivery suite and have blood grouped and saved prior to delivery. Uterine atony is by far the commonest cause. Basic resuscitation steps should be taken initially; however, in major post-partum haemorrhage, active management should take place with vaginal examination identifying the cause, and if low tone of the uterus is identified, bi-manual compression can be performed. In other cases, patients can be taken to theatre to look for a possible cause, such as a laceration which can be stitched. In extreme cases, > 10 L of blood can be lost and the patient requires massive transfusion. In these circumstances, often uterine artery embolisation or hysterectomy are needed to cease the bleeding. Post-partum haemorrhage is usually avoided with active management of the third stage of labour with administration of oxytocin.

# A¹²

1. External urethral sphincter and pelvic floor exceeds the detrusor pressure. **(1)**
2. Increasing parity, menopause, perineal trauma in childbirth, surgery, chronic cough, obesity, chronic constipation. **(1)**
3. Cystocoele: prolapse of anterior vaginal wall containing bladder. Residual urine may cause dysuria.

   Rectocoele: prolapse of the posterior vaginal wall containing rectum. Patient may need to manually reduce in order to defecate.

   Stress incontinence: urine leak occurs when intra-abdominal pressure raises, e.g. sneezing, coughing, laughing. **(1 mark for each, max 3 marks)**
4. Diabetes, urinary tract infection. **(½ a mark for each, max 1 mark)**
5. Urodynamics. **(1)**
6. Avoid caffeine, pelvic floor exercises, weight loss, avoid alcohol, avoid drinking immediately before bedtime if nocturia is prominent, bladder training to increase time between voiding, avoid blackcurrant drinks, avoid fizzy drinks. **(1 mark for each, max 2 marks)**
7. Antimuscarinics such as oxybutynin, tolterodine, solifenacin. **(1)**

Prolapse can cause much distress and embarrassment for women who suffer from it. A prolapse is when weakness of the supporting structures allows pelvic organs to protrude into the vagina. It is strongly although not exclusively associated with pregnancy and childbirth with perineal repair. Many women present post-menopausal as surrounding supports have reduced further. Third-degree uterine prolapse is where the uterus is outside of the introitus and can cause ulceration and ureteric obstruction. Symptoms include a mass sensation, dragging, sexual dysfunction and difficulty with defecation. Manual reduction may be needed in order to pass stool. Non-surgical candidates can be treated conservatively with pelvic floor physiotherapy, weight loss, smoking cessation, vaginal oestrogens and ring or shelf pessaries, which sit in the vagina and support prolapsed tissue. Surgical prolapse management involves excision of loose tissue and resuturing to strengthen support. Hysterectomy can be considered for severe prolapse.

# A13

1. Inability to complete full sentences, resp rate ≥ 25 breaths/minute, tachycardia ≥ 110 bpm, peak flow 33%–50% predicted. **(1 mark for each, max 3 marks)**

2. Arterial blood gas, chest X-ray, ECG, sputum culture. **(1 mark for each, max 2 marks)**

3. Ipratropium bromide, prednisolone, hydrocortisone, magnesium sulphate, aminophylline, terbutaline. **(1 mark for each, max 2 marks)**

4. Leucotriene receptor antagonist (e.g. montelukast), theophylline. **(1 mark for either)**

5. Check inhaler technique, check compliance with medications, consider use of spacer, allergen avoidance, increase exercise. **(1 mark for each, max 2 marks)**

Acute severe asthma is severe asthma that has not been controlled by the patient's current medications. Common triggers are infections and known allergens. History should include asking about previous hospital admissions, ITU admissions and current drug history to gauge the severity of their asthma. Peak expiratory flow (PEF) is a simple way of measuring the severity of the current episode and forms part of the criteria to determine the severity of the attack. The criteria for diagnosing acute severe asthma have been listed above. Signs of life-threatening asthma include PEF < 33% best/predicted, bradycardia, hypotension, exhaustion, confusion, cyanosis and a silent chest. Notify your senior team and ITU if a patient is exhibiting any of these signs. An arterial blood gas should be taken to ensure there is not severe hypoxaemia, type 2 respiratory failure or severe acidosis, and a chest X-ray should be arranged to rule out a pneumothorax. The majority of cases of acute severe asthma can be managed with oxygen and nebulised salbutamol and ipratropium bromide. If symptoms do not improve with these measures, oral B agonists, magnesium sulphate and/or aminophylline may be considered. Steroids are often given orally for minor attacks, but may be required intravenously if severe. Infections should be treated with appropriate antibiotics.

# A¹⁴

1. One in 25. **(1)**
2. Sweat test, genetic testing. **(1 mark for each, max 2 marks)**
3. Recurrent chest infections, pneumothorax, bronchiectasis, pulmonary hypertension, aspergillus, nasal polyps. **(1 mark for each, max 2 marks)**
4. Pancreatitic malabsorbtion. **(1)**
5. Cirrhosis, intestinal blockage leading to increased constipation, obstruction and intussusception, increased reflux. **(1 mark for each, max 2 marks)**
6. Excessive amounts of fat present in the faeces. **(1)**
7. A, D, E, K. **(½ a mark each, max 2 marks)**

Cystic fibrosis is a common autosomal recessive disorder. About one in 25 Caucasians are carriers. The mutation affects the cystic fibrosis transmembrane conductance regulator gene. Ultimately, the disturbance to the sodium-chloride channel leads to viscous secretions. These thick secretions lead to pancreatic insufficiency, raised sodium content in sweat, and lung diseases. Treatment involves a multidisciplinary approach supporting respiratory problems and the nutritional needs of the patient by supplementing digestive enzymes, vitamins and a high-calorie diet.

# A¹⁵

1. Chemicals, electricity, radiation. **(2)**
2. Thermal injury to the airway may lead to airway oedema and therefore obstruction, so expectant intubation may be necessary. **(1)**
3. Wallace rule of nines, Lund and Browder chart. **(1)**
4. Superficial burns: pain, blisters, erythema, brisk capillary refill.

   Full-thickness burns: painless, no blisters, white/grey/black, absent capillary refill. **(2)**
5. 4 × body weight (kg) × body surface area (%) = volume of Hartmann's solution (ml) to be given over 24 hours. **(1)**
6. Half the volume should be given over 8 hours and the other half over 16 hours. **(1)**
7. Infection, dehydration. **(2)**

The majority of burns are minor and heal with no complication. However, major burns require urgent assessment and should be rapidly transferred to an acute medical facility. Initial management should be via an ABCDE approach with particular attention to airway assessment and management by an anaesthetist, fluid resuscitation, adequate analgesia and the prevention of hypothermia. The areas of the body affected by burns should be irrigated and dressed appropriately. All complex burns should be referred to a specialist burns centre for further management. In patients who have inhaled smoke, the possibility of carbon monoxide poisoning should be considered.

# Bibliography

Collier J, Longmore M, Turmezei T, *et al. Oxford Handbook of Clinical Specialties*. 8th ed. Oxford: Oxford University Press; 2009.

Cook J, Sweetland H. *Crash Course: surgery*. 1st ed. St Louis, MO: Mosby Ltd; 2000.

http://emedicine.medscape.com/

www.gpnotebook.co.uk

Impey L, Child T. *Obstetrics and Gynaecology*. 3rd ed. Chichester: Wiley-Blackwell; 2008.

Kumar P, Clark M. *Clinical Medicine*. 6th ed. London: Elsevier Saunders; 2005.

Longmore M, Wilkinson I, Turmezei T, *et al. Oxford Handbook of Clinical Medicine*. 7th ed. Oxford: Oxford University Press; 2007.

National Institute for Health and Clinical Excellence. *Hypertension: clinical management of primary hypertension in adults: NICE guideline 127*. London: NIHCE; 2011. Available online at www.nice.org.uk/guidance/CG127

www.patient.co.uk

# Index

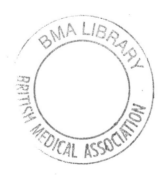